For Marie,
With love, always,
Joy
13ᵗʰ Jan. 1996

JOURNEY TO WHOLENESS

Morris Maddocks has been Adviser for the ministry of health and healing to the Archbishops of Canterbury and York for 12 years and is an assistant bishop in the diocese of Chichester. He and his wife Anne founded the Acorn Christian Healing Trust. He is the author of *The Christian Healing Ministry*, *The Christian Adventure* and *Twenty Questions About Healing*.

... "We were called on a journey to the wholeness that is in God alone ...

Love is the motive power behind a̲ for it is rea̲ ̲ ̲ ̲e of the Sp̲

Wholeness ... ultimately is a journey into God for He alone is that perfection. The Christ who makes all things new, including us, is the Alpha and the Omega, the beginning and the end of our journey. P. 8.

Also by Morris Maddocks

The Christian Healing Ministry (SPCK)
Twenty Questions About Healing (SPCK)

Journey to Wholeness

Morris Maddocks

TRI∆NGLE

First published 1986
Second edition 1995
Triangle
SPCK
Holy Trinity Church
Marylebone Road
London NW1 4DU

ACKNOWLEDGEMENTS

Biblical quotations come from the New International
Version of the Bible, copyright © 1978 by the New
International Bible Society, first published in Great Britian
in 1979, and are used by permission.

The quotation from Little Gidding, Four Quartets
by T. S. Eliot is reproduced by permission of
Faber & Faber Ltd.

British Library Cataloguing in Publication Data

Maddocks, Morris
Journey to wholeness.
1. Pastoral medicine   2. Pastoral psychology
I. Title
265'.82   BV4337

ISBN 0-281-04852-5

Typeset by Pioneer Associates, Perthshire
Printed and bound in Great Britain by
BPC Paperbacks Ltd
Member of the British Printing Company Ltd

Contents

Contents

Foreword

This book has grown out of Anne's and my experience 'on the Way' in the past two years. We are grateful for the constant encouragement we have received from very many people, especially from fellow-travellers on the Way in all the churches and in Medicine. Much that has been distilled here has come out of our conversations together, privately or in seminars, when we have shared experiences. Many will recognize themes of my lectures in which I have tried to point to the large dimensions and purpose of the journey.

I constantly return to the journey as the best model to guide our thinking about Christian healing. It distinguishes healing from curing at the outset, and enables one to see how God is in charge of the whole operation and is able to use even the misfortunes and dis-ease as part of his overall plan of wholeness for the world community and each individual within it. It is this plan which Jesus Christ came to further, and he who is the Way calls us to follow him on this journey to wholeness as his people of the Way.

The vision for our work and witness is that all will travel together as the healed and healing community. The purpose of the journey is a healed creation, not just a collection of new individuals. The whole is greater than the sum of its parts and that is why, under God, it is a journey to wholeness. The healing of the churches and of the caring professions is therefore of prime necessity, as well as the healing of society and nations. There is much business to be done on the journey. Pray we may listen more intently to our marching orders.

Anne and I want to thank Richard and Anne Holmes for their work on a preliminary manuscript and June Hall who has once again painstakingly and cheerfully typed the completed manuscript; also the publishers. We also thank all who have had us and the writing of the book in their prayer. We gratefully dedicate it to our Trustees and colleagues of the Acorn Christian Healing Trust and all with whom we have worked during the past ten years in the Churches' Council for Health and Healing and at St Marylebone Parish Church.

St Peter's Day 1985   *Morris and Anne Maddocks*

Preface to the Second Edition

Anne and I are grateful to Triangle Books and in particular the editor Naomi Starkey for the decision to publish a new edition of this little book. Since writing this during the first years of my work as Adviser to the Archbishops and in the early years of Acorn, we have travelled a long way in many senses. But I believe that the idea of the journey is the best figure of speech to apply to the Christian Healing ministry and I am thankful that over the last 10 years, since the book was published, the Christian Healing ministry has made its own journey in to every department of the churches' life and witness. Let us all remember that the purpose of our travelling on this journey is to co-operate with our Creator in His continuing work for a healed creation.

Conversion of St Paul 1995   *Morris and Anne Maddocks*

1

Preparing for the Journey

'In the beginning God'. But also 'In the end God'. We cannot ask for anything less as the parameters of our journey. We are in search of wholeness. Can it be set in any other context than that of the totality of God and his redeemed creation? The Creator was in the beginning and saw that his Creation was good. Only at the end will that perfection be attained once more when God is all in all and all things return to their pristine perfection.

The healing of individuals has, therefore, to be seen in the light of the reconciliation of creation to its Creator. This is the purpose of our journey to wholeness. In the meantime all healing is inevitably partial while this process of integration is undergone.

Process and journey are good metaphors for our understanding of healing and health, which we have tended to believe, along with many other things in our contemporary life, are instantly available and are ours to possess by right. Rather they are given us, often through striving and suffering. And when we think we have them in our grasp, they are not finally possessed since in our humanness we are still subject to sickness, accident and death. The important factor, however, about the journey is that we should set out.

What is health?

It has been claimed that Alternative Medicine is the fastest growing industry after that of computers. Certainly health is now 'big-time' as people do their daily jog, count their calories and spend thousands of pounds in the mushrooming health food shops. The media are also in on the act, or perhaps they promote it: no day passes without a newspaper article or television programme on health.

Many have attempted definitions. I always liked the one I first heard from Dr Sydney Evans: Being in tune with the song the Creator is eternally singing.[1] Most people leave God out of their search for health, and yet Carl Jung said he could not bring healing and health to anyone without first restoring to them their religious sense. This rational world of ours has neglected the spiritual element of a person's well-being. Our National Health Service, however, began on the right lines when it insisted on making provision for the spiritual needs of hospital patients. There is a dimension to our health beyond the undoubted expertise of the medical profession.

This is brought home by a case history from a hospital chaplain's notebook. He tells of a typical (sadly for our time) Saturday night in an accident ward. There had been a particularly bad car crash involving four teenagers. When they were brought in, their lives hung by a thread. Four medical teams had to work hard to keep the youngsters alive.

The chaplain prayed at each bedside and then left the ward lest he got in the way of the doctors and nurses. He procured the names of the next of kin and began to telephone their homes. The first parent told him he had dialled the wrong number and put the phone down, causing him to ring again. The second told him firmly that his daughter was upstairs in bed. He asked the father to check this; of course she couldn't be found. The third abused the chaplain for bothering him and told him if he had got his son he could keep him as he had never been anything but a load of rubbish. The fourth set of parents could not be contacted as they were out at an all night party.

During the next weeks, as the medical skill combined with the innate healing powers in those four bodies to restore them to health, the chaplain tried to get alongside them. Then they were discharged as 'healthy' young people once more and went 'home'. The chaplain was saddened and yet not totally surprised when one of them returned a few weeks later having been involved in another car pile-up.

What is health in this case? And for that matter what was 'home'? I asked myself these questions when I had to visit the accident wards in our local hospital on another Saturday night. The young son of one of my priests had been knocked down by a car just outside his house. He never regained consciousness. There in the ward were several young people in various states of disarray, causing the medical teams to work very hard. Like the chaplain I tried to pray, keeping out of the way and then went outside. An ambulance-man was bringing in someone else and I muttered something about what we do to each other with our motor cars. I have never forgotten his reply — and its implications: 'Quiet night tonight, sir; and at least those in there are alive.'

Obviously health is far more than the absence of disease. From these experiences alone we learn it has to do with our relationships, being loved, having a purpose in life, being true to ourselves and others.

The biblical ideas

Relationships were very important to the well-being of man

3

in Hebrew history. The most important relationship was with God, and the Hebrews thought of it in corporate terms. It was the community that must maintain this relationship in good order and individuals enjoyed this relationship — which was often seen in terms of marriage — through the tribe. The relationship was therefore expressed either in terms of fidelity, or of obedience to the Law of God given through Moses and adherence to God's word as expressed by the leaders or prophets. Disobedience or unfaithfulness by the tribe led to lack of well-being and further states of sin and infidelity. There was, in fact, a lack of health when the relationship was severed and the covenant that bound it was broken.

The relationship with one's neighbour was also vital to individual and corporate health. 'Thou shalt love thy neighbour as thyself' was the second commandment of the Deuteronomic law. The equilibrium of the tribe was upset if individuals were not in harmony. Health meant good relationships with God and man.

When Bishop Stephen Neill talked about health and the Bible he used to add two more relationships which he considered should be in good order for a healthy way of life: with oneself and with the soil. The first is implied in the second commandment — to love one's neighbour *as oneself*. Care for one's own being and total well-being is an act of worship to one's Creator. We do not serve God well if we fail to care for our own health, especially our spiritual health. Nor do we give worship to our Creator by polluting or destroying his creation. For our health it is important that we relate to the soil and to all creation, particularly the animal kingdom.[2]

These relationships were all considered important for the well-being of God's people. The Hebrew word for this healthy state, with well-ordered relationships, was *shalom*, which means much more than our usual translation of peace. In fact it is impossible to translate into one English word since it covers total well-being, prosperity, bodily health, contentedness, good all-round relationships and even salvation or perfection and fulfilment. Above all it was the gift of God which could be received only in his presence. It was in fact 'being in tune with the song the Creator is eternally singing', being totally healthy in body, mind and spirit. And this healthiness was expressed in community; it was a corporate well-being. The *shalom* of any individual was for the good, the *shalom*, of the whole. In fact *shalom* came to the individual from God through the community. The biblical world was an interrelated world, a network of relationships in which everyone and everything affected each other and related to the whole. It is this kind of world that the mystics have known down the ages. It is this world that the new sciences, especially physics, are opening up for us again today. And that is the radical change which hopefully will transform our era from an individualistic existence with an insistence on selfish rights into a wholistic[3] existence with a motivation towards mutual obligations. It is more likely to be a world of *shalom* when mankind has undergone the transformation. It will be a world that knows to a greater degree the things that belong to its health. The scriptures will help us in this process of change, provided we do not use them as a blueprint (for every age is different) but listen and learn from their wisdom. We shall then be listening to the voice of God and back on course, forging a relationship with him, which is the priority on any journey to health and wholeness.

What is healing?

It is more than curing, with which many confuse it. It is rather a process, which may take a long time, that leads to health and wholeness. It will therefore affect every part of us. Most people think of it only in regard to the body, physical healing. That is obviously important to each one of us. But we have to open our eyes to a larger view of life. We also have a mind, emotions and a spirit within us. We therefore need mental healing, emotional healing and spiritual healing. Yes, all of us are in need of healing — total healing.

Gradually we are learning about the marvellous and complex piece of creation that is 'me'.[4] Truly we are 'fearfully and wonderfully made' and even now much of the mystery of the human personality remains unfathomed. What we do know is that all the many strands that go to make up a human being are interwoven, interlocking and interrelated. This means that the chemistry of my body can affect the disposition of my mind or spirit, while the spiritual part of me can raise or depress my physical or mental state. If my body is sick the question to ask is, why? It may not be entirely the fault of 'brother ass'. It may not even be my 'fault' at all: I may be reflecting the dis-ease in my family or in society. We are fairly complex characters! When we think of healing, therefore, we have to take a wide canvas. The whole situation, the environment and all that impinges on the life of the person, even from the past, has to be taken into consideration, because our healing is a microcosm of the total healing which God is preparing for his creation.

Mercifully we are not without assets. Our body is equipped with a powerful immune system and every part tends to heal when damaged. We also have spiritual resources because we are made in God's image. Unfortunately, just as the body's immune system can malfunction when under stress or overtired, so our spiritual resources can decay through lack of inspiration and through neglect. Most of us need to go on a course of spiritual jogging in order that our innate powers of healing can be fully motivated. The atrophied remains of many people's spiritual systems are largely responsible, I suspect, for much of their ill-health.

Healing is the 'good' thrust in creation. The writer of the first creation story in Genesis continually comments, 'God saw that it was good'. Here is the healing element in all parts of God's creation. If you cut down a tree, it tends to sprout upwards again. If you cut your finger, it tends to heal. Healing is the 'natural' resource in all creation. It is God's power for good which he has shared with all his creation. It has been advanced by the sending of his Son, Jesus Christ, by whose stripes we are healed, by whose cross/resurrection the world has been reborn and in whom our healing can be fulfilled. He is 'the Way', the light on our journey to wholeness.

A new vision of healing

Through the incarnation of his Son, God initiated the task of putting the world to rights. As we shall see, Jesus encapsulated his vision of a healed creation in terms of the Kingdom of God, his Father reigning in every part of his creation. He 'earthed' this vision supremely in his healing ministry, as he went about 'healing people who had all kinds of disease and sickness' (Matt. 4.23; 9.35 etc.). He met people exactly where they were, at their point of need. And he met every need, not just their physical need, but their mental anguish or spiritual disability also. His healing was truly wholistic. He lifted people out of the mess in which they found themselves, sometimes through no fault of their own, and set them on their way again, their journey to wholeness. He gave them a new vision for life.

As we set out we shall try to keep the purpose of our journey in mind. It is a journey towards wholeness which ultimately is a journey into God, for he alone is that perfection. The Christ who makes all things new, including us, is the Alpha and the Omega, the beginning and the end of our journey. Let us begin with two pilgrimages, both of which will take us back into the history of man's search for wholeness, before we return again to the new vision being offered to contemporary pilgrims.

2

A Biblical Pilgrimage:
Healing and Wholeness in
the Old Testament

The Bible is a record of the God who calls. He calls people and nations to join him on a journey. Because God is at the head, it is a journey to wholeness.

Abraham is the first historical figure called to embark on this journey. He is called to leave his father's house in utter obedience. In one of the early visions on the journey he is told: "'Look up to the heavens and count the stars — if indeed you can count them . . . So shall your offspring be." Abram believed the Lord and he credited it to him as righteousness' (Gen. 15.5–6). The word used for believing here comes from the same root as that from which we derive our word 'Amen'. The ancients had come to realize that the touchstone of their being blessed on their journey was their willingness to set out. They must say their 'Amen' to the call to set out. To travel was to go with God. Their 'Amen' was therefore an act of faith in the wholeness to which God was calling them, the response of faith to God's will to heal and bless them.

The wholesome relationship between God and man is expressed in the word righteousness, indicative of a behaviour and mutual respect in keeping with a creative and healthy relationship. The journey will impart an awareness of the living God and will therefore be a healing and maturing experience.

As the patriarchal journeys continue we see this

relationship being forged ever more strongly as constantly the 'Amen' of faith is given in response to God's call to set out on the adventurous journey of life. The journey to Moriah to sacrifice Isaac must have been prefaced with a costly 'Amen', but set out Abraham did, and his reward was the revelation that 'the Lord will provide', the name he gave to the place. The journey to find a wife for Isaac was similarly blessed and tells us something of the healing which man seeks in his search for the perfect partner. Jacob's journey to find a wife who might bring him the healing he never knew in his own home was blessed all along the way. At Bethel (*house of God*), the name he gave to the place where he had his famous dream of the ladder, God assured him that there would be a continuous line of communication between them on his journey of life, and indeed for ever: 'All peoples on earth will be blessed through you and your offspring. I am with you and will watch over you wherever you go, and I will bring you back to this land. I will not leave you until I have done what I have promised you' (Gen. 28.14–15). Little wonder he felt himself to be at the gate of heaven. His line of descent would lead to the birth of the world's Saviour and Healer. It is of interest that in the morning he anointed with oil the stone on which he had rested. Oil was supposed in primitive belief to renew the vitality of the indwelling god. This could be interpreted as a prophetic act, since the disciples of the Lord's Anointed now use sacramental oil as a sign of the healing Christ's (*the Anointed's*) indwelling and presence with the sick. This and the ladder are symbols of our need for constant spiritual communication with the Lord through sacrament and prayer in all our travelling.

Jacob was to have another encounter during the night on his journey home many years later. In what was possibly a wakeful dream, Jacob wrestled with the angel at Peniel (*the Face of God*). It may have been his subconscious mind trying to convince his conscious mind, full of anxiety and foreboding about meeting his brother on the morrow, that all would be well. God not only removed the anxiety, effecting a deep healing between the brothers on the following day, but he also gave Jacob a blessing beyond his dreams: 'Your name will no longer be Jacob, but Israel (*he struggles with God*), because you have struggled with God and with men and have overcome' (Gen. 32.28).

How frequently our own anxieties are washed away in the tide of God's love, bringing in greater blessings than we could have ever anticipated. We constantly underestimate the divine potential! Frequently, also, an act of reconciliation such as the one in which Jacob was engaged, can open up opportunities of healing for the whole community. Such initiatives bring unforeseen blessings on the journey to wholeness.

Some of the most moving stories in the Old Testament, are to be found in the Joseph saga. Like his father Jacob, Joseph was also a dreamer. The dreams of his youth were likely to shatter family harmony, but how true they were in the event. His dreaming gave him the skill of interpretation, a gift that was not only to save him from a lingering death in prison, but also to be the salvation of Egypt and, more especially, of all his father's house. His sojourn in exile was to be most fruitful and bring healing to many.

Again the theme of the whole story is reconciliation, and the climax is reached in one of the most moving chapters in all literature when Joseph reveals his true identity to his brothers. The dream of his youth found fulfilment, but of far greater significance for Joseph was the working out of God's purpose through the events of his life's journey: 'Do not be distressed and do not be angry with yourselves for selling me here, because it was to save lives that God sent me ahead of you . . . God sent me ahead of you to preserve for you a remnant on earth and to save your lives by a great deliverance' (Gen. 45. 5,7). Joseph was quite convinced that God had guided his life in order to preserve the life of his family and bring a new wholeness to their life together, as well as preserving their posterity. Their God was a God who heals and saves.

The patriarchal sagas have sounded the recurring melodies in the biblical symphony. The God who calls out his own on the journey of life works from darkness to light, doubt to faith, slavery to freedom, death to life. We shall hear them again and again, but never more so than in the mighty events of the Old and New Testaments, described in one word which preserves the idea of the human journey to wholeness — Exodus (*way out of*, and so, *going forth*). It is the word used by Luke in the account of the Transfiguration when Jesus conversed with Moses and Elijah about his imminent work of salvation and healing (Luke 9.31).

In the Old Testament, it became the great act of God in history on behalf of his people Israel. It was not merely an heroic escape by a captive people, but an act of deliverance by their God, through which a whole nation, clean contrary to the inclination of the majority and against the might of a powerful king and nation, was led out of a slave labour camp, snatched from the path of their pursuers and set on their journey to new life. It is hard for us, through rationalist eyes, to discern the ultimate significance of this event of salvation history, but for the Jews it was the watershed in the life of their nation, the supreme point of departure in their history, *the* mighty event of the Old Testament. In Christian eyes, it was the foreshadowing event of the second

Exodus: the cross/resurrection of Jesus which was the mighty act of God's deliverance in the New Testament and the departure point for the history of the Christian Church.

The Exodus was the point at which Israel first encountered God as a nation. It was a corporate religious experience which welded the Israelites together and conferred on them a national unity. The unlikely birthplace of this revitalized nation was the slave labour camps of Rameses II who, like other rulers we have known in our time and throughout history, projected the shadow side of his nation on to an unpopular ethnic group. His elaborate construction schemes in the Nile delta were largely built by the sucessors of Joseph and his brethren. It was out of the darkness of this slavery that God summoned his people to journey into the freedom of being his children, with the supreme purpose of being the instrument of his will on the world stage. The catalyst of this memorable part of the salvific journey was to be Moses.

Here is another melodic theme that constantly repeats itself during this whole symphonic journey: God calls men and women, usually out of sickness or slavery or persecution from which he delivers them or heals them, to be instruments of his will and to further his purpose on the journey of life. Moses was a perfect example of God's call-for-a-purpose. In answering the call he became one of the greatest religious leaders of all time. He uttered his 'Amen' to the call to set out, though at first with some reluctance. (Don't we all?) His miraculous escape via an 'ark' among the bulrushes seemed to demonstrate beyond all doubt that God's hand was upon him, the ark being a symbol of salvation.

It is possible that the almost miraculous preservation of Moses' life at the time of his birth was the archetypal symbol of new hope which kindled the dying embers of an apparently hopeless nation.[1]   Here was the necessary image which stimulated the hidden potential of life that lay dormant in both Moses and the Israelites. It is like the shaft of light that providentially flashes across one's path when the going seems impossible and hope is waning during some of life's crises. It is a warm glow that is sufficient to rekindle the dying fire in us and set us on life's journey once again, 'strangely warmed'.

This glow was fanned into flame by Moses' call at the burning bush, fire invariably being a biblical symbol of the presence of God. The event therefore underlines the fact that Moses received his call from God. But how was God to be described? Undoubtedly he was the God of the Patriarchs: Abraham, Isaac and Jacob; but how was he to be named to a new generation? In what way could Moses communicate to a spiritless and depressed people that God was still active on their behalf? It is a question that faces every generation of religious leaders who seek to help people forward on the journey. God is of unchangeable power and might, but each generation responds to him differently because we can only glimpse one small part of his character. Moses knew how important it was in primitive religion to know the deity's name before cultic relations could be initiated. He therefore saw how essential it was to establish such relations between God and his people if he was to have any hope of leading them on the journey. He had the insight of a true pastor! It is primarily the relationship between the people and their God which it is vital to establish, not that between the people and their priest or leader. Wholeness is a gift of God's grace.

The name was also important because it indicated character, and Moses knew the Israelites to be a practical people. They were bound to ask, 'Who? Of what nature? Of what potential, is this God?' People are still asking that question today, and how vital it is to demonstrate that the God we proclaim is mighty in *deed* as well as in word. The Kingdom can only be proclaimed by preaching and *healing*.

Moses was given a significant answer: 'God said to Moses, "I AM WHO I AM." (or "I WILL BE WHAT I WILL BE"). This is what you are to say to the Israelites: "I AM has sent me to you." God also said to Moses, "Say to the Israelites, The Lord, the God of your fathers . . . has sent me to you." This is my name for ever' (Exod. 3.14ff.). The name 'the Lord' in verse 15 is a translation of the Hebrew consonants YHWH which is connected with the verb 'to be', hence the name I AM. In fact, the reading of the future tense is to be preferred — I WILL BE WHAT I WILL BE. Here is the true character of YHWH, or Yahweh as he is now to be known with the Hebrew consonants filled out. The God who will be what he will be is always on ahead. He promises to be with Moses always, as he will also be with his people. Yahweh is the God who will guide history and lead his people on their journey and reveal himself to them continuously. In the pitfalls of the road, in the problems that face them on the way, in their joys and sorrows, Yahweh their God, our God, will be there. That's the only reason it can be called a journey to wholeness: God is always with us on the way and on ahead calling us on. In Jesus he is revealed as the Way. It is to the very beginning of the Israelites' journey to wholeness of nationhood that this distinctive faith and unique conception of God can be traced. Even the eighth-century prophets, who more than anyone helped to form the Jewish theology, all point back to the Exodus as the moment of the birth of Israel's unique faith in the God who is active in history, constantly guiding his people whom he has called to be a light for the nations. Yahweh is essentially the God-on-ahead.

The call of Moses was one of the most significant issued by God to man in religious history. It was to leave the security of family and home, like Abraham, to return to share the hazards and hardships of his own people in captivity, and then to undertake the Herculean task of liberating his people from bondage and leading them on the greatest journey, certainly of Old Testament times, through the wilderness to the Promised Land. God had in fact asked him to preside over the birth of his own nation. Little wonder Moses was diffident. But God was faithful to his promise and Moses never let his gaze wander from Yahweh, the God who will be what he will be. The Israelites for their part, despite incessant grumbles, instinctively knew they had a leader who walked with God. It was that knowledge which kept them going on the journey.

We have already hinted at the important place of symbol in our lives; images that speak to our deep consciousness and evoke the latent powers within us. The whole of the Exodus event is redolent with symbol. *The plagues* that Moses and Aaron visited on the Egyptians to persuade them to let the Israelites go, speak of the groaning and travailing of creation, nature's echo of the mighty event the Creator is bringing to pass. *The Passover,* to commemorate the passing over their houses of the angel of death with the sign of the blood of the lamb on their doorposts; *the feast of unleavened bread,* so named because they had to go out in haste and could not wait for the bread to be leavened, thereby symbolizing a complete break with the past; *the dedication of the firstborn* to Yahweh, recalling the 'night of watching by the Lord', to bring them out of the land of

Egypt (Exod. 12.42). For Christians, these symbols — the blood of the lamb, the bread, the night of watching — became even more meaningful in the light of Christ's passion and the events of that particular Passover. Highly significant too is the similarity of the symbols surrounding the first and second Exodus and of the journey of God's people in each mighty event towards salvation and wholeness. The essential factor in both is that God is in the journey, guiding at each step, calling his people forward from on ahead, in command of the whole situation, working out his vast purpose for the world he created. What a lesson for our own journey!

For the Jews there has never been a stronger conviction that this was so than in the whole Exodus event and particularly in the crossing of the Red Sea. The Exodus was the constitutive event of their history, paralleled by the 'ab urbe condita' of Rome and the 'anno Domini' of Christianity. Moses' hymn of thanksgiving (Exod. 15.1 – 18), probably expanded from the ancient fragment of the Song of Miriam (v.21), is echoed throughout the Old Testament, pointing to Israel's conviction that at this point in her history, Yahweh had laid his hand upon her and so commissioned her to be his people. The crossing of the Red Sea (and the reader must discern there are three main sources describing the event, and most events throughout the Exodus) is looked upon as the great deliverance and is regarded as the proof of God's will and power to save. It is a theme we meet throughout the Bible in all the journeys of God's people.

Let us pause at this point to notice a few of the details. First, the 'outstretched arm' with which God has promised to redeem his people (Exod. 6.6). Symbolic of God's power to save and heal, that constant biblical theme we have just

17

discerned, it also signifies adoption, commissioning, identification with and blessing. This is the divine act which gives
meaning and significance to the laying on of hands which the
Old Israel as well as the New (the Christian Church) has
used ever since, as when rabbis chose their pupils for
another year (adoption); or the apostles ordained elders
(commissioning); or the sins were laid on the scapegoat
(identification with); or hands were laid on the sick
(blessing, though here there is a coming together of all the
various strands). The hand that was stretched out to effect
the mighty deliverance of the Exodus will not be held back
from identifying with, and touching, our infirmities. His arm
is indeed stretched out still, upon all our journeys.

Then, the pillar of cloud and fire (Exod. 13.21). Here we
find the outward symbol of Yahweh, 'I WILL BE WHAT I WILL
BE', the guiding and guardian God, who is always on ahead
preparing the way. Fire and the cloud are both symbolic of
the divine presence, and assured the Israelites that Yahweh
was with them on their journey. It is good to stop and ask
ourselves the spiritual question, what constitutes the cloud
and the fire on our own journey? It is a question that may
convert us from always working *for* God, which too
frequently means doing what *I* think God needs done in his
world and in his Church, to working *with* God. It is all *his*
work.

Yet again let us observe the words of command given to
the Israelites at this momentous and crisis point in their
journey. The first was given by Moses: 'Do not be afraid.
Stand firm and you will see the deliverance the Lord will
bring you today. The Lord will fight for you; you need only
to be still' (Exod. 14.13–14). It is a great word for all
journeys of God's people. When we come to a crisis in our

18

lives our normal reaction is to fuss, to become anxious, to think about it over and over again until our minds become a whirl, rendering clarity of thought and sensible action impossible. Moses knew better; he nipped their anxious grumbling in the bud and lifted their eyes from themselves to the God-on-ahead-who-saves. How essential to stand and stare, to fill our minds with all the positive good that is happening in the whole creation, so that our hearts and minds are lifted to the Creator and to pondering on his creative and saving work. 'You need only to be still.' There is a time for prayer, as well as prayer being all the time.

There is also a time for action, which should always come after prayer. (How often we reverse the process!) So to a people stilled, quiet and watching, God was able to speak and the people were able to hear: 'Tell the Israelites to move on' (Exod. 14.15). Here too is a word for all our journeys. For the invariable tendency of too many of God's people is to go back in their pilgrimage, either totally, giving up the whole venture, or to a safe period of their life, thus preventing the maturing process and aborting the journey to wholeness. Elsewhere I have written about *The Christian Adventure* and it still seems to me that life is meant to be seen in terms of adventure. 'The Holy Spirit, who is the spirit of Movement and Adventure, is always calling us to look forward, and if we are sensitive to his pressures, we find he is always leading and driving us on.' This was the experience of the Israelites after they had stood still. They came to realize that the way to tackle the journey to wholeness was to move on, if they wanted to attain to the full salvation of Yahweh, the God-on-ahead.

And so they came to the wilderness, the place where God educated his people. If the crossing of the Red Sea waters was, as it were, the baptism of Israel, God's firstborn people, the wilderness saw the nurturing and education of the new-born nation. Hosea (11.1−4) describes this period so well:

When Israel was a child, I loved him,
    and out of Egypt I called my son.
But the more I called Israel,
    the further they went from me . . .
(Yet) it was I who taught Ephraim to walk,
    taking them by the arms;
but they did not realize
    it was I who healed them.
I led them with cords of human kindness,
    with the ties of love.

'They did not realize it was I who healed them'; and yet this was to be the message of the first revelation on this part of the journey. The signs and wonders did not cease with the events that accompanied the Exodus: the sign and revelation immediately following the great deliverance (the writer notes it was three days!) was, I believe, to be continually meaningful in the journey of God's people. It has particular significance in demonstrating that God will supply all their needs. It is a sign which the people of God have never taken seriously enough.

Marah, which means 'bitterness' because of the water found there, was the setting. After the sweetening of the water, the writer tells how the Lord revealed himself in a particular role − as healer: 'If you listen carefully to the voice of the Lord your God and do what is right in his eyes, if you pay attention to his commands and keep all his decrees, I will not bring on you any of the diseases I brought on the Egyptians, for *I am the Lord, who heals you'* (Exod. 15.26). The recognition of, and faith in, Yahweh as sovereign and only Lord, implying complete obedience and commitment to his word, carries with it the word of assurance that he alone is the source of all healing, as well as the word of promise that he will exercise his healing power on behalf of his people. The promise of healing was made conditional on obedience to the word of the Lord. 'If you will listen carefully . . .' Health in the Old Testament was dependent on a life lived in obedience to God's commands. There could be no wholeness for the individual or the nation if either lived in apostasy. Health had to do with all departments of life and for the Hebrews the relationship with Yahweh was the most important. This is the lesson relentlessly hammered home throughout the wilderness journey: obey God and live free from dis-ease; disobey God and dis-ease is bound to follow. The fatal plague followed the rebellion of Korah (Num. 16); snakes poisoned the people when they spoke against God and Moses (Num. 21); the remedy, the serpent on a pole, was an early essay in homeopathic medicine and is now the emblem of the medical profession.

Obedience produces a positive condition of wellness, an inner consciousness of being God's own. It leads to a feeling of being in tune with the song the Creator is eternally singing. The hearing of God's word, with its implication of obeying, as in the Latin *audio*, is the direct road to health and, as Dr S. I. McMillen showed in his book *None of These Diseases*, is a powerful preventive force against many ills. This demand for corporate obedience was met by a positive response on the part of the Israelites in the covenant at Sinai.

In one way the Sinai covenant was not entirely new to the

21

Israelites. In the covenant with Abraham (Gen. 15.18) God planned to save the world through a particular community which Abraham had been called to found. But no one person or nation could be the instrument of salvation until they themselves had experienced such salvation, had known the saving power of God at first hand. Abraham was saved at the eleventh-and-a-half hour from sacrificing his own son; Israel had now experienced the mighty deliverance of the Exodus. The scene was therefore set for the ratification of this relationship, a relationship marked by trust and obedience and issuing in a missionary vocation to the world. The terms of the covenant were the Ten Commandments (Exod. 20. 1–17), which were to be the covenant sign of God's own people, a pattern which could mould their lives on common spiritual principles and be a permanent reminder of the saving power of God shown in the Exodus. At their very root lies the authority of God: 'I am the Lord your God' (Exod. 20.2), a reminder that man will never attain journey's end under his own steam, without the divine help of the God who heals and saves. The covenant relationship conveys the recognition by man that he is a creature dependent on his Creator and that the word addressed to him may often be a word of challenge and uncomfortable to hear.

But what was the real purpose of the journey through the wilderness? It is well summarized by a later writer: 'Remember how the Lord your God led you all the way in the desert these forty years, to humble you and to test you in order to know what was in your heart, whether or not you would keep his commands. He humbled you, causing you to hunger and then feeding you with manna, which neither you nor your fathers had known, *to teach you that man does not live on bread alone but on every word that comes from the mouth of the Lord'* (Deut. 8.2,3). This was the great lesson God taught his people on the wilderness journey. It must have been particularly important because the lesson went on for forty years! Indeed it seems an impossibly difficult lesson for mankind to learn, even over four thousand years. 'Not on bread alone, but on every word that comes from the mouth of the Lord.'

The wilderness, however, is a good classroom. It is a vast open space, open to all possibilities. Open to disasters as well as blessings, open to hope as well as danger. Like the Israelites, whenever we go through the wilderness section of our journey, we too are open to hope, the promise of better things to come. We are also open to danger; perhaps we may fall by the wayside, either from the exterior difficulties we encounter or from the inner fears and forebodings. For in the wilderness the person we shall meet most often is our true self! And that is an encounter that can spell either hope or danger.

It is at this point that the 'not on bread alone' lesson is so important. We need to perceive and hear what is coming from the Lord's mouth. And first that means the standing still which Moses enjoined upon the Israelites on reaching the Red Sea, *in order to hear* the word from the Lord's mouth that followed: 'Tell the people of Israel to move on.' It is essential to move forward from where I am in order to know more of myself and more of God, the always-on-ahead-God who revealed himself as Yahweh, 'I WILL BE WHAT I WILL BE'. And as we move forward, the danger and the hope will fall into place, as part of the maturing process, part of our journey to wholeness. Both are essential. The Bible does not simply speak of danger. If so, our faith would be reduced to a protection-from-danger religion. Nor does it only speak of hope. If so, our faith would merely be a happy-ending religion. The Bible views the journey of life as a meeting with both danger and hope, a crisis situation. But in the wilderness God is always calling us to look forward, beyond the protection-from-danger religion, beyond the happy-ending religion, to HIM. God is saying, 'Trust ME. Come and see (Jesus' word to Andrew) the vastness of my love for you. Wait upon the word from my mouth and stop worrying about the bread. TRUST ME.'

For most of us this will be a lesson of full forty years' duration, possibly longer into eternity. It takes some learning. But the wilderness is the place that slows us down sufficiently to be able to hear 'every word that comes from the mouth of the Lord'. Too often the noise of our rush and speed, of our busy-ness and selfishness, prevents us from hearing the word of the Lord. Or perhaps we rationalize away the intuitive promptings we hear and then ignore them. Life is too often all bread, all materialism, all a search for power, all puff like some of the blown-up bread of today. It is hard to hear the voice of the Lord in the busy streets and motorways of our crowded lives.

But the wilderness, the place of storm and tempest in our life because we are open to all possibilities, the place of danger and yet of hope, slows us down to a listening speed[2] and we find we can hear again, just as an illness or tragedy can stop all our busy-ness at a stroke. The key factor is then to ask the spiritual question — why? 'What is this sudden event in my life teaching me?' 'What is God teaching me through it?' The wilderness, the place where we can only walk — there are no motorways or high speed trains — not only enables us to ask such a question but gives us the

24

possibility of hearing an answer. The wilderness is the classroom of salvation, a vital part of our journey to wholeness. It is constantly lit by the presence of God. The pillar of fire by night and the cloud by day are just as real experiences for God's people today as they were for his people in the time of Moses.

> One the light of God's own presence
> O'er his ransomed people shed:
> Chasing far the gloom and terror
> Brightening all the path we tread.

Virtually all the remainder of the Old Testament, indeed of all Jewish history, is lived out in the afterglow of the Exodus. The Decalogue used to be repeated as the people's response of faith to the recitation of Yahweh's mighty act of deliverance of his people in the Exodus. The keeping of the Torah was the continuous outworking of that obedience demanded of the nation so delivered. Judges and Kings attempted to lead the people in worship and obedience to the God-on-ahead; some did so with greater success than others. The Psalmist continually sang of the healing God of the Exodus 'who only does great wonders'.

It was left to the eighth-century prophets to clothe their God with understandable attributes and make him more knowable, even approachable. The first Isaiah was overwhelmed with the holiness of Yahweh and saw him as demanding a like holiness in his people. Amos served the righteous God and prophesied in the northern kingdom to a people that largely rejected the demand for a correspondingly righteous way of life. Micah saw Yahweh as the just God, and inveighed against contemporary injustices among

25

his people. Hosea, sometimes called the St John of the Old Testament, was the first to see Yahweh as a God of love, and through the tragedy of his own marriage was led to perceive the utter faithfulness of his God who goes on loving his people despite their unfaithfulness to him.

All of them warn both kingdoms — Israel in the north and Judah in the south — of the consequences of their disobedience and unfaithfulness to their God who led them to freedom through the waters of the Red Sea. Above all it is Jeremiah who sounds the final warning note and has to live through the destruction of the nation and its 'city of peace', Jerusalem. The remnant goes into Exile, and this experience of suffering and deprivation is cathartic and ultimately therapeutic.

The Exile experience is interpreted by two great prophets — the second Isaiah and Ezekiel. They discern the hand of 'the Lord who heals' in this whole traumatic episode of Jewish history and see that it will lead to a triumphant return to a restored wholeness, worthy to be compared with the deliverance of the Exodus. The music of Handel's *Messiah* has made the prophecies of Deutero-Isaiah (see chapter 40) some of the best known and best loved words in the Bible. The Good Friday liturgy has made some of his other prophecies equally well known — the passages usually named the Servant Songs. In these remarkable pieces of prophetic writing Isaiah became the first person to hold out the possibility of cosmic redemption and healing through innocent suffering. The Gospel writers were quick to connect these prophecies with Jesus and with the cosmic implications of his innocent suffering on the Cross. For instance we read in the first Servant Song:

> I will keep you and will make you
> to be a covenant for the people
> and a light for the Gentiles,
> to open the eyes that are blind,
> to free captives from prison
> and to release from the dungeon
> those who sit in darkness.

(Isa. 42.6–7)

If this fitted the person of Jesus, the third and fourth Servant Songs are almost eye-witness accounts of his Passion:

> I offered my back to those who beat me,
> my cheeks to those who pulled out my beard;
> I did not hide my face
> from mocking and spitting.

(Isa. 50.6)

and again:

> He was despised and rejected by men,
> a man of sorrows and familiar with suffering.
> Like one from whom men hide their faces
> he was despised, and we esteemed him not.
> Surely he took up our infirmities
> and carried our sorrows,
> yet we considered him stricken by God,
> smitten by him, and afflicted.
> But he was pierced for our transgressions,
> he was crushed for our iniquities;
> the punishment that brought us peace was upon him,
> and by his wounds we are healed.

(Isa. 53.3–5)

Here is one of the many great high points of the Old Testament. The dawning awareness suddenly comes over the speaker that this despised human being, passed over in his suffering and total weakness, is the very earthen vessel God is using to bring healing to mankind. The Servant's totally innocent suffering 'brought us peace' (*shalom*, the nearest Old Testament idea to health and wholeness), and his innocent wounds brought healing to mankind. This is a unique insight in the Old Testament that was to be fulfilled in the New. It was not the strength of God's Servant that would avail to effect such a redemptive healing of cosmic proportions: rather it was his weakness. The fact that 'by his wounds we are healed', is an experience put into words which unfolds a whole new revelation. The path to wholeness cannot be attained solely through our own effort, but through someone called by God to suffer on our behalf. It is by his stripes, not our own.

This fourth Servant Song ends with the words:

> For he bore the sin of many
> and made intercession for the transgressors. (v.12)

This act of intercession is more than words. It is acted out in deed also, as the Servant offers his very suffering as the act of intercession. Here is the word/deed theme found in the person of Moses and fulfilled in Jesus, the second Moses, picked up by Isaiah and lived out in the person of the Servant in these prophecies. He 'made intercession' by offering his own life, expressive of the true meaning of the word, 'to take up your stance in between God and man'. This work is perfectly fulfilled in the healing ministry and teaching of Jesus, which reached its climax in the *deed* of innocent suffering on the Cross.

28

This word-and-deed methodology is taken up in a remarkable prophecy of the third Isaiah, the prophet who saw the return of the exiles from Babylon. It is all the more remarkable since in Luke's account of the ministry, Jesus took the passage for his first sermon at Nazareth, applying it directly to himself:

The Spirit of the Sovereign Lord is on me,
　　because the Lord has anointed me
　　to preach good news to the poor.
He has sent me to bind up the broken-hearted,
　　to proclaim freedom for the captives
　　and release for the prisoners,
to proclaim the year of the Lord's favour
　　and the day of vengeance of our God,
to comfort all who mourn,
　　and to provide for those who grieve in Zion —
to bestow on them a crown of beauty
　　instead of ashes,
the oil of gladness
　　instead of mourning,
and a garment of praise
　　instead of a spirit of despair.
They will be called oaks of righteousness,
　　a planting of the Lord
　　for the display of his splendour.

(Isa. 61.1 – 3)

In the Lucan passage, only verse 1 is quoted which, after silence, is followed by Jesus' comment 'Today this scripture is fulfilled in your hearing' (Luke 4.21). Certainly Jesus filled the role of the Lord's Anointed — the Christ, which is the same word. Certainly he came to proclaim the good news, and his stance was always among the poor. His work of healing was especially of benefit to the broken-hearted, the blind (a better reading than prisoners) and all held captive by 'the world, the flesh and the devil'. The special blessings, however, seem to be reserved for the mourners and those who grieve, those who have had some rough deals in life. They will receive beauty for ashes, the oil of gladness (the name happily given to the oil of healing used by the Roman Catholic laity) for mourning, a garment of praise for a spirit of despair.

This last is a true word of healing. Praise changes the direction of our life, reversing the downward pull, dispelling the oppression from the shadow side of us. It changes us at the centre, because our body immune system is put into top gear and all our reactions are made positive. C. S. Lewis must have experienced this disclosure moment because he once said, 'Praise is inner health made audible.' There would be more positive health and constructive living in our world if people would don 'the garment of praise'. Such people would be the 'oaks of righteousness', the sort of solid and dependable people who have sorted out their relationship with God and with one another. People who spend time in praising God are indeed 'a planting of the Lord for the display of his splendour'. Being attuned to the Lord constantly, they reflect his glory. It was a happy choice of a word of Scripture to herald the beginning of Jesus' ministry.

The final word in the Old Testament comes from Malachi, 'the Messenger', who prophesied in the fifth century BC, after the return of the exiles and after the reforms of Ezra. He looked forward to the day of the Kingdom when creation would be healed: 'For you who revere my name, the sun of righteousness will rise with healing in its wings' (Mal. 4.2).

The day of the Lord would be a day of vindication, a day when all relationships would be perfectly healed, heralding a new dawn of history in which creation would attain to its destiny of wholeness in the Lord. The end of our journey comes when God is all and in all. 'The Kingdom of God is creation healed.'[3] In the meantime the pilgrimage continues.

3

A Medical Pilgrimage

'The cure of a part should not be attempted without treatment of the whole. No attempt should be made to cure the body without the soul . . . The great error of our day in the treatment of the human body is that physicians first separate the soul from the body.' This was not the utterance of some avant-garde doctor or theologian of the present century, relevant though it may seem to the contemporary scene. It was in fact written by Plato around 380BC. He was inveighing against the materialistic attitudes of the healing profession of his day. He considered they were wrongly applying the teaching of Hippocrates. In short they were not truly wholistic in their treatments.

One of the treatises in the vast Hippocratic corpus is entitled *Airs, Waters and Places*. It seeks to show how the air we breathe, the water we drink and the topography of the land all have some effect on our general health. We have been slow to rediscover such truths in our time, but credence is being given once again to the effect of 'non-medical' factors upon the body's immune system. I think it may be unfair to blame the medical profession entirely for such tardiness. Because of the advances of science the general public has been conditioned to expect some magic formula or panacea for its ills and itself has been slow to realize that the root causes of illness may be capable of treatment and especially prevention much nearer home. It is hard to convince a general public served by a national health service that each of us is responsible for our own health. After all, my body belongs to me (a Christian would affirm to God) and not to the state!

The conditioning of science can be illustrated by considering what happened in the very beginning. If you asked an astro-physicist he might start by telling you it all began with a very hot and outsize bang. As a result, the fragments are continuing to shoot through space at immense speeds. The universe is therefore one vast and ever-expanding whole, evolving continually.

If you asked a theologian, he might refer you to Genesis chapter 1, explaining it is not an eye-witness's account, but a subsequent writer's reflections on evolution. He might also refer you to the Prologue of the Fourth Gospel: 'In the beginning was the Word and the Word was with God, and the Word was God. He was with God in the beginning.'

It may be a sad comment on our educational system, but I would hazard a guess that the majority of young students would say the astro-physicist was right. We have been conditioned to think, even to write theology, with that 'scientific' mentality. The fact is that both the astro-physicist and the theologian are right and both their insights are necessary to our understanding of the whole. The astro-physicist was attempting to say something about origins — when? how? what? The theologian was attempting to say something about meanings — why? And that is essentially the spiritual question in life. The astro-physicist was answering in terms of time, the theologian in terms of beyond time, timelessness. For an understanding of man, both these dimensions are essential.

There is a move throughout the medical profession today to reach beyond the totally scientific view and consider all factors. This has been brought about partly by the amazing advances in medical science, bringing in their wake ever more moral and ethical decisions. But those very discoveries of science have also shown that there is no ultimate answer provided by science to all the problems of human health care. Man has another dimension that has to be recognized and brought into all considerations of therapy.

In fact these very advances in science have been made possible by a particular mode of thought that has dominated scientific thinking for the past 300 years since the age of the Enlightenment. It is usually referred to as Reductionist. Descartes ('*Cogito ergo sum*' — I think therefore I am) helped to establish the primacy of logic and reason, separated from and independent of external influences. He viewed the human body as a machine, after the fashion of a clock: 'My thought compares a sick man and an ill-made clock with my idea of a healthy man and a well-made clock.' Since then science has largely viewed the body as a machine. The Cartesian method was to analyse and reduce the difficulties into as many parts as possible, examining each part separately. This reductionist view has influenced much of medical research and the practice of clinical medicine. At the time, Descartes , and shortly after him Newton who, with his brilliant grasp of mathematics, completed the scientific revolution of the seventeenth century, effected a significant liberation for the human spirit. It was, however, to exchange one straitjacket for another, to pass from dogmatic religion to an equally dogmatic science. William Blake saw the truth of the situation and painted God and Newton measuring the universe with a compass. He also foresaw the advent of holism when he was moved to write:

To see a world in a grain of sand
and a heaven in a wild flower

34

Hold infinity in the palm of your hand
And eternity in an hour.

Nevertheless the analytic and reductionist method, with its belief in the rational approach to human problems, has been the cradle of thought and education, of research and clinical medicine, until recent times. It has led to very great discoveries in individual fields as specialization has increased more and more. It has been the matrix of our upbringing, of our way of life, of the other sciences and disciplines, including theology. But great changes are on the way. Who or what are the catalysts?

Modern physics has played the role of midwife to a new world view. In contrast to the mechanistic Cartesian view of the world, the emerging world view might well be called a systems view and is characterized by such words as holistic, organic, ecological. 'The universe is no longer seen as a machine', wrote Fritjof Capra in his formative book *The Turning Point*, 'made up of a multitude of objects, but has to be pictured as one indivisible, dynamic whole whose parts are essentially interrelated and can be understood only as patterns of a cosmic process.' It is the interrelatedness and interconnectedness of the universe, one whole system to which billions of smaller systems contribute and play their indispensable part, that is important for the understanding of life today. One scientist underlined the total significance of relationships when he said that they should form the basis of all definitions. An object should be defined solely by its relations to other things. 'An elementary particle . . . is in essence a set of relationships that reach outward to other things.' Even the observer is involved in these relationships and his very observation influences the course of the whole. Truly we are part and parcel of each other and of the dynamic creation in which we have evolved.

The systems view of life is essentially spiritual and is seen to harmonize at many levels. The mystics have known this level of experience for hundreds of years as they underwent other states of consciousness and felt an affinity with the universe. We ourselves may have experienced a momentary consciousness of spiritual oneness with the universe as we hit the perfect golf stroke or contemplate a great work of art, as we pray or watch the splendour of a sunset or sunrise. At such times we have known we are part of a great whole, that we are in harmony with the universe or with the God who creates it. It has been a 'disclosure moment' of eternal significance. Teilhard de Chardin essayed to integrate into an ordered system and coherent world view his scientific knowledge, his theology and his mystical experiences. Rejected in his lifetime by science and religion, both held in the net of a constricting Cartesian world view, his ideas may now gain wider credence in the emerging systems or wholistic world view and will make a necessary contribution to the evolving harmony between scientists and mystics and all who seek to take a wholistic view of life.

All this will have immense consequences for our attitudes to health and healing and to our approach to the treatment of disease, and for the way we essay our journey to wholeness. We shall, however, not be embarking on a totally new voyage of discovery. A wholistic approach to our subject will have an affinity with many traditional views. For instance, among primitive tribes the shaman was usually the political leader, religious guru and doctor all rolled into one. He was a powerful figure. The shamanistic attitude to illness was that it indicated some disharmony with the cosmic order, because it was held, in a similar way to modern physics, that human beings were part of an ordered system. So much for progress! The shaman would therefore first sit down with the elders of the tribe when called to a case of sickness, and question them about relationships with the environment and within the tribe. The remedy would emphasize the restoration of balance and harmony with the natural and spiritual world and with all relationships. Possibly Western scientific medicine, while making immense discoveries concerning the biological mechanisms and physiological processes that produce symptoms of disease, has neglected this emphasis on the sociocultural and spiritual context of illness.

Psychotherapy is of course attempting to redress the balance. Shamanistic healing rituals often sought to raise unconscious hurts and conflicts to a conscious level, along the lines of modern psychotherapeutic practice. It is interesting that centuries ago the shamans used such 'modern' techniques as group sharing, dream analysis, hypnosis, guided imagery and psychodrama. The shamans also placed a far greater emphasis on the collective and social aspects of therapy, so that the patient would be healed into the community once again. Much of our therapeutic practice has been too individualistic, even in the Church. 'The universal shamanistic view of human beings as integral parts of an ordered system', writes Fritjof Capra, 'is completely consistent with the modern systems view of nature, and the conception of illness as a consequence of disharmony and imbalance is likely to play a central role in the new holistic approach (to health).'[1] It is also not far from St Paul's doctrine of the Church as the Body of Christ, in which 'if one part suffers, every part suffers with it' (1 Cor. 12.26).

Greek antiquity also made its contribution to health-

37

giving insights. It has chiefly contributed to the holistic model in that healing was considered to be essentially a spiritual phenomenon. Greek religion was of course polytheistic and its background was mythology rather than very serious theology. However, an interesting fact is that the two goddesses associated with Asclepius, the god of healing (the symbol of western medicine is a serpent coiled round the Asclepian Staff), represent facets of the healing art still valid today: *Hygeia* (health, from which we get our word 'hygiene') was concerned with the maintenance of health, what we might call today 'preventive medicine'; while *Panakeia* (Panacea, all-healing) was concerned with remedies, and so therapy. In any holistic approach it is important to keep a balance between both these aspects of health care. The present medical model has tended to emphasize the latter, while the churches have tended to neglect the former through an over-emphasis on the cure of souls.

It is of course Hippocrates who represents the culmination of Greek medicine and who has had the most lasting influence on current medical science and practice. It was he (or his school, because the Hippocratic corpus probably owes its origins to many hands) who laid the foundations of modern scientific medicine. The breadth of his vision, however, has not always been maintained. *Airs, Waters and Places,* one of the books of the Hippocratic corpus, has already been mentioned as showing how health comes from a state of balance among environmental influences. He also recognized the healing power of nature and stated that the role of the physician was to act as an attendant or assistant to these natural forces (Greek *therapeuein,* 'to attend', from which is derived our word therapist), creating favourable conditions in which the healing can take place. The Hippocratic tradition, with its emphasis on these aspects of therapy as well as its emphasis on the interrelation of body, mind, spirit and environment, has more than any other laid the foundation of the modern holistic approach to medical treatment.

One further influence was the Chinese tradition, which had its roots in the shamanistic tradition and was shaped by both Taoism and Confucianism, the two principal philosophical schools of the classical period. Again the idea of balance is fundamental. The two archetypal poles are central and the entire universe is considered as being in a state of dynamic balance, with all its components oscillating between them. The poles are called *yin* and *yang*, the former being more conscious of the environment, the latter of the self. The *yin* inclines to intuitive knowledge, the *yang* to the rational. In this way *yin* is supposed to be more feminine, *yang* more masculine. Because rational knowledge is linear, focussed and analytic, it tends to be fragmented. Intuitive knowledge on the other hand tends to be synthesizing, holistic if you like, deriving from the meaning of the Greek *holos* 'whole', referring to an understanding of reality in terms of integrated wholes. The present emphasis in medical care is moving towards the *yin*.

Starting from this fundamental balance in the universe, Chinese medicine saw the healthy person and the healthy society as integral parts of a great patterned order, while 'the Chinese notion of the body as an indivisible system of interrelated components is obviously much closer to the modern systems approach than to the classical Cartesian model'.[2] The approach to health care was always made in terms of accurate diagnosis which would determine areas of imbalance, especially with the environment, followed by a prescription of as mild a therapy as possible in order to restore that balance and harmony. It can be seen that all these therapies are designed to tackle the sources of ill-health, rather than merely alleviating the symptoms. One encouragement to the doctor to get to the bottom of things quickly was that he was only paid while the patient remained in good health! Payment ceased at the onset of an illness.

All these ancient concepts of health care are being given mileage once again as we come to a more wholistic view of things. Many health practitioners use what is known as the wholistic approach and examine all the factors relevant to the patient, especially the environment, relationships, diet, life-style etc. Of course it must be said that a majority of the medical profession has probably used this method in normal clinical practice all the time. However, it seemed good to a large number of doctors of all ages and traditions to state this publicly in 1983 by forming the British Holistic Medical Association. They place the emphasis on whole-person medicine, whether according to orthodox or complementary (a better word than alternative) medical practice, and 'incorporate into their map some of the more recent scientific discoveries that enhance our understanding of how we function as human beings', such as the insights of modern physics and the concept of field force in human functioning and stress. They are seeking to resurrect the art of healing and are aware of the spiritual causes of illness as well as spiritual remedies. Here are some of the basic, universal principles of holistic medicine, which, as the reader will note, have their origin in some of the traditions that have been referred to already, but which are now being supported by the discoveries of the new science. I shall set them out exactly as Dr Patrick Pietroni gave them in his inaugural address to the British Holistic Medical Association:

1. The human organism is a multi-dimensional being, possessing body, mind and spirit, all inextricably connected, each part affecting the whole and the whole being greater than the sum of the parts.
2. There is an interconnectedness between human beings and their environment which includes other human beings. This interconnectedness acts as a force on the functioning of the individual isolated human being.
3. Disease or ill-health arises as a result of a state of imbalance, either from within the human being or because of some external force in the environment, and by environment I include the family.
4. We each possess a powerful and innate capacity for healing ourselves or bringing ourselves back into a state of balance.
5. One of the primary tasks of someone entrusted to heal, be he doctor, priest or acupuncturist, is to encourage the self-innate capacity for healing of the individual in distress.
6. This primary task can often be better accomplished through education than through direct intervention, whether that intervention be penicillin, surgery or a homoeopathic prescription.
7. To enable him to accomplish his task effectively the healer needs to be aware of his own multi-dimensional levels of existence and have some expertise and ability in achieving a state of balance and harmony within himself. (Physician, heal thyself.)

Some Christians would want to add or subtract a little, particularly by an emphasis on the source of, and reason for, that interconnectedness and innate healing property — the Creator of whose creation we are privileged to be part. The awareness, however, of the spiritual cause of much disease, especially because of an imbalance of chemistry within the individual and more importantly of external relationships — with God or with fellow human beings — which frequently may cause chemical imbalance or malfunction of the immune system or of other parts of the human body or mind, is greatly to be welcomed by all who take seriously the fact that 'we are fearfully and wonderfully made'.

Advances towards a more holistic approach are being made in all specialities of medicine. A more integrative and humanistic approach to cardiovascular disease has been pioneered by Dr Peter Nixon of Charing Cross Hospital among others. His famous 'human function curve' demonstrates how an abnormal amount of effort and needless stress impairs our normal performance to a point of fatigue and exhaustion. If persisted in, such a life-style will lead to ill health and eventual breakdown. When expressed in such plain terms, it is hoped that coronary care will be shifted back a few stages, from intensive care to the preventive stages, far more frequently. This will require a massive drive to educate the public. Perhaps the doctor of the future will increasingly live up to his name, which means 'teacher'.

Another cardiologist, Herbert Benson of Harvard University Medical School, has pioneered a way of dealing with environmental stress and written about it in his great little book *The Relaxation Response*.[3] To the traditional explanations for the prevalence of hypertension — inappropriate diet, lack of exercise, family disposition — Benson adds a fourth, environmental stress. His remedy is the Relaxation Response which has always existed in religious teachings. His thesis is well researched with ample quotations from Eastern and Western mystics and contemplatives. For the meditative exercise he sees four essential elements: 1) a quiet environment; 2) a mental device such as a word or a phrase which should be repeated constantly; 3) the adoption of a passive attitude, which is perhaps the most important of the elements; and 4) a comfortable position. The prescription is once or twice daily for ten to twenty minutes. The physiological and psychological changes in a person who adopts the Relaxation Response are abundantly obvious.

Of course, this is nothing new in a religious setting. The ancient religions of the East and Christianity, especially in the West, have been teaching such methods of meditation for centuries. What is new is to have it prescribed by doctors of scientific medicine to cure the body. It seems that we should 'persevere in prayer', not only for our salvation but for our health! What happens is that a daily 'dose' of meditation or contemplative prayer slows down and balances the body chemistry, which in turn acts as a preventive measure against stress and anxiety, enabling us to cope better when problems and crises occur, thus ensuring that our body immune system is not put under tension or resulting risk. We do not become tired or exhausted so quickly and life is lived on a much more even keel. I suspect we also become nicer to know! I also believe that as we hear more about stress, increasingly we shall hear more about meditation and prayer in treatment and hopefully less about sedatives. The latter are far too expensive in any case, and thousands of pounds could be saved by the NHS in our country if doctors and priests worked together, holding simple meditation classes. To my way of thinking it would more significantly remove much of the anger and violence from society, which in a curious way seems to be perpetuated in part by constant reliance on drug therapy.

The essence of holistic medicine is that, because it seeks to treat the whole person, it does not merely attempt to improve health levels by treating symptoms but by examining the root causes of disease. The researches of Dr Malcolm Carruthers of the Bethlem Royal and Maudsley Hospital into stress, tension and heart disease were summarized by one meditation master in the words: 'Rage and fear are the masters of heart failure.' His researches have proved to him that the practice of religion 'can lessen the impact of stress on one's life and reduce dependency on tranquillizers, sleeping pills etc . . . Both the people who "die well" and those who make the best recovery are often those who have either had or develop strong religious beliefs.' It seems obvious that unless the spiritual part of a person's make-up is developed and brought to bear on the therapy, it will not necessarily meet with success, certainly not permanent success. Possibly the overall sickness that afflicts the human race is spiritual sickness, and spiritual sickness requires spiritual remedies. Doctors who take a fully wholistic approach, that is, treat the whole person, will inevitably find this is so, and that is why we shall see more spiritual treatment in order to get to the root of the matter. It is for these reasons that someone like William Temple felt it wrong that doctors and priests worked entirely apart from each other. A man generations ahead of his time, he saw the vital necessity of whole person medicine.

All this has implications for both medical and theological training. The medical schools rarely give sufficient emphasis to the spiritual part of man and its contribution to healing. De Vries drew attention to this neglect of the spirit in medical training in 1981, and Malcolm Wetgler reported from his conversation with students that they felt one element to be 'totally lacking —

44

represented by the Quaker statement: "There is that of God in Everyman"'. It was felt to be lacking not only in the teaching concerning treatment, but also in relationships, even in medical school! My own experience with young doctors on their vocational courses confirms this. They have told me that the spiritual side of man was not touched on in their curriculum at medical school. I suppose the main occasion when this element of our make-up is encountered in clinical practice is when patients lose the will to live. Most doctors realize that they then require a priest for their clinical colleague. We must work together so that this realization comes at an earlier stage in the treatment.

Many people regard health as something outside their own understanding, as something conferred upon them by the expertise of the doctor or the drugs he prescribes. They tend not to see it as something to which they can contribute. Whole person medicine insists that not only must the whole person be considered and involved in the healing process — body, mind, spirit, emotions, bio-energy — but the whole person must himself or herself contribute to that process. The medicine of tomorrow will depend much more on the willingness of the patients themselves to be involved in their own healing process. The discoveries of the new physics which demonstrate that we are all interconnected and part of each other underline the fact that this is the way to wholeness and health.

I want to end this chapter with a plea to all health practitioners. Turn again to, and learn again from, the healing example of Jesus Christ. It has been affirmed that Jesus is as much the father of western medicine as Hippocrates. He spent one third of his ministry in healing the sick. His methods were invariably wholistic. He always went to the roots of the person's disease. He treated people as people, as his brothers and sisters, as fellow children of his Father in heaven. Their life was infinitely precious and he made it abundantly plain that he wanted them well. He 'snorted' at some forms of sickness, angry that his Father's creation was being disfigured. Constantly the Gospel writers report how he healed all who came to him. It was his very nature to heal, and in this he manifested supremely the grace and truth of God. And when he healed he saw the making of a new, whole person as a sign of the breaking in of the Kingdom of God, a sign that through him God was putting the world to rights, that his Father's reign on earth was already manifesting itself in a re-creation, a new wholeness of life. Furthermore, when he commissioned his disciples and sent them out to proclaim the Kingdom, he insisted they did it not only by word of mouth but by deed also, by healing as well as preaching; in a word, by making men and women whole, as the heavenly Father meant them to be.

Can medicine ignore these facts? Can it be called truly holistic without taking on board something of the legacy of Jesus of Nazareth as well as that of Hippocrates of the Island of Cos? Can the contribution of Christian spirituality be omitted from whole person medicine? Or, put the other way round, can the contribution of Christian healing be omitted from a wholistic theology?

There are many wonderful legacies of the Enlightenment for which we must praise God. On the debit side, it has tended to reduce our spiritual vision resulting in a compartmentalization of disciplines. One result of this has been the privatization of religion and medicine. Both need to break out of this straitjacket and catch a wider vision of their role: to teach man to attain to the fullness of life God intended. Only thus can he co-operate with his Creator in putting the world to rights for the benefit of humankind and for the glory of God. In Christ such a new creation can be accomplished, for such is the healing on offer. And this underlines the need for the church and medicine to journey together as the healing community in which man can be enabled to move forward on his journey to wholeness.

4

In Search of a Vision

A stout seat which has weathered many winters stands by a fishpond in a corner of the garden at Chartwell. Here Churchill sat for hours, gazing across the Weald of Kent. The glorious landscape, stretching endlessly into the distance, proved to be a creative canvas for his thoughts during his wilderness years.[1] His frequent contemplation of the scene led him to see visions and dream dreams. His artist's eye became matched by a developing religious sense. It was a blessing for this country that he was given sufficient space in which to contemplate so that he had a vision not only of his own destiny but of the nation's.

A person of vision develops a sense of timelessness and spaciousness. Timelessness leads to a knowledge of occasion, the right time, which in fact is the New Testament meaning of time, *ho kairos*. Spaciousness gives a sense of freedom which institutional life seeks to inhibit. It was Bishop Donald Coggan who reminded us in his book *Convictions* that the very root of the name Jesus contained the idea of spaciousness. People whom Jesus calls into his service need space to move and grow in order to realize their destiny. Their pilgrimage as people of vision, their journey to wholeness, must have a timeless and spacious quality about it. After all, their vocation is to see God, and see him reigning.

There was a timeless quality about the life of Jesus. His earthly life was lived in the shadow of eternity. There were thirty years of virtual silence in preparation for three years

48

of ministry. He invariably gave himself space. A long while before day he went out alone into the hills to commune with his heavenly Father. His life was lived in a contemplative stillness which allowed him to be a person of vision and realize his destiny. 'Crowds of people came to hear him and to be healed of their sicknesses. But Jesus often withdrew to lonely places and prayed' (Luke 5.15–16). Not even the pressures and demands of real human need deflected him from his own spiritual journey. There is a lesson here for a church when it can only see the proclamation of a social gospel as the reason for its existence.

Jesus encapsulated his vision in terms of his Father's sovereign rule over the world. He knew his vocation to be the setting to rights of his Father's creation. This vision of the world recreated he expressed in terms of the Kingdom of God. 'The true manifestation of the Kingdom of God', in Hans Kung's memorable phrase, 'is creation healed'. All the energy and earthly striving of Jesus of Nazareth was directed to that end. The Kingdom of his Father, his Father's coming to rule in all parts of his creation, was the vision that remained undimmed in the consciousness of Jesus, even on the cross. In fact it was precisely through the cross, through entering the gate of death, that the vision eventually came to be realized: 'When thou hadst overcome the sharpness of death: thou didst open the Kingdom of heaven to all believers.' It is the vision of the Kingdom that all of us who follow Christ need to recapture today. May it become increasingly meaningful as this new era unfolds.

What lies behind the teaching of Jesus on the Kingdom of God?

As a background, it is helpful to note the way the concept was used in apocalyptic, especially in the period immediately preceding the coming of Jesus. Chiefly it was used in two ways: the first, to express 'the expectation of God's decisive, eschatological intervention in history and human experience'; the second, 'in reference to the final state of the redeemed to which God's intervention in history and human experience is designed to lead'. Jesus' teaching reflects both of these usages, that is, both the present and the future hope.[2]

As regards the first usage, Jesus, at the very outset of his ministry, challenges the people by proclaiming that God's decisive intervention in history is imminent: 'The time has come . . . The kingdom of God is near. Repent and believe the good news' (Mark 1.15). He commissions his disciples to bear the same unrelenting message (Matt. 10.7; Luke 10.9,11), which includes as its visible expression the healing of the sick. It is not therefore surprising to find that Jesus tells his hearers that God's intervention can be seen in his exorcisms (Matt. 12.28; Luke 11.20). What was entirely in the future according to apocalyptic expectation can here and now be experienced by the individual who benefits from the healing activity of Jesus and his disciples. As Norman Perrin says: 'The experience of the individual has become the arena of the eschatological conflict.' The exorcisms and healings of Jesus and his disciples are evidence that the forces of evil are being rendered powerless. God has asserted his reign. The ancient Kaddish Prayer and the Lord's Prayer are being answered. His Kingdom is at hand.

This seems to be the thrust of two further sayings, the first in Matt. 11.12 (cf. Luke 16.16): 'From the days of John the Baptist until now, the kingdom of heaven has been forcefully advancing, and forceful men lay hold of it.' It is a difficult saying and open to various interpretations, but what Jesus seems to imply is that a new stage in man's consciousness began with John the Baptist, a new paradigm shift, in which there is a greater awareness of the Kingdom's presence. As is customary in totally new situations, the anger in man swells up and he revolts against change when he sees familiar landmarks threatened. This is especially true in the context of established institutions. But the very fact that this is happening is a sign of the Kingdom's presence, itself a sign that the eschatological conflict is taking place. Acts of violence against the Kingdom will continue until God's final victory, though that victory has been assured by the victory in the cross/resurrection of Jesus.

The other saying can be found in Luke 17.20–21: 'The kingdom of God does not come with your careful observation; nor will people say, "Here it is," or "There it is," because the kingdom of God is within you.' This is the strongest assertion of the intervention of God's kingly rule actually taking place in human experience. It marks a return to the prophetic understanding of history in which God acts in certain historical events and through them challenges the nation or individuals to respond. Here is the ultimate challenge to the individual, when God acts within that person. The Kingdom of God *within* is the ultimate in human experience: it is a foretaste of the vision of God.

We must return now to the second usage of the term 'Kingdom of God' – in relation to the final state of the redeemed. God's intervention in history and human experience, which we have so far been discussing, is the necessary preliminary to this final state. Jesus' constant use of the term 'Kingdom of God' to express the final goal as well as the intervening events in which God acts, gives a coherence and wholeness to the vision he came to bring.

In the Beatitudes, Jesus delineates the values of the

51

Kingdom and presents to his disciples a vision of life lived in the end time. It will be noticed how the values that are counted as 'normal' in society today are completely turned upside down. It is the poor, the mourners, the meek, the hungry, the merciful, the pure, the peacemakers and the persecuted who are singled out for blessedness. They will be signs of the Kingdom, for such characteristics are pointers to the fact of God's reign within a person. For them, God has made all things new, and worldly standards have ceased to count. These are the standards which, lived out by Christ's followers, turn the world upside down. It is the reversal that is inherent in all Jesus' teaching: 'Many who are first will be last, and many who are last will be first' (Matt. 19.30). It is of interest that this summary occurs in the context of teaching about the end time, 'the renewal of all things'.

Close examination of much of the Sermon on the Mount will also reveal its claim to be a recipe for health in this life; an essay, as it were, in preventive medicine. Jesus' insistence that we reject all anxiety, for instance, would, if obeyed, improve the health of any nation by fifty per cent. The British in particular seem to be a nation of worriers. Hence our over-large consumption of drugs.

The Beatitudes also are roads to health. How therapeutic it is to mourn and grieve. Much sickness comes upon us because we do not allow ourselves time and opportunity to go through this necessary part of bereavement. Or again, to be merciful: resentment, vindictiveness, persistence in anger or vengeful thoughts are also sure recipes for cardiac disease or other 'killers'. Or again, to be peacemakers: for people who create harmony and well-being in all their environment are also people who are healed inwardly and have peace in their own hearts. How we need to maintain this vision, this reflection of the new values from the future Kingdom of God! For our present purpose, however, we are considering the final state of the redeemed in the end time.

Another saying of Jesus in this regard is Matt. 8.11 (cf. Luke 13.29). Here Jesus pictures a great multitude coming from all parts of the world to join the Patriarchs at the heavenly banquet 'in the Kingdom of heaven'. It is a common biblical illustration, in which eating and drinking symbolize the vision of God. The symbol of a banquet in the end time is used in apocalyptic writing and is very much part of the teaching of Jesus. We meet it at the end of the Last Supper, when Jesus tells his disciples he 'will not drink again of the fruit of the vine until that day when I drink it anew in the kingdom of God' (Mark 14.25 and parallels). For Christians, the healing conveyed to them by Christ in the eucharist is a foretaste of the heavenly banquet.

There are also many passages relating to entering and receiving the Kingdom of God. Entry will be gained only by those whose righteousness surpasses that of the establishment (Matt. 5.20) and who receive the vision of God's Kingdom with childlike obedience and trust (Mark 10.15) and do the Father's will (Matt. 7.21). For those whose life centres on the amassing of wealth and who trust in riches, entry to the Kingdom will be hard (Mark 10.23–31). It will be easier for the outcasts of society than for them (Matt. 21.31). Entry into the Kingdom will also require severe self-examination and self-analysis (Mark 9.47).

All this indicates how Jesus used the Kingdom of God in this sense of the end-time quite frequently in his teaching. Constantly in his use of the term he emphasizes the activity of God and, true to the prophetic teaching, he views history as the milieu in which God's activity is revealed. The purpose of this revelation is for the salvation of humankind, for it procures for man the perfect relationship with God. In short, the Kingdom of God, the establishment of God's reign, makes possible the vision of God.

Because of these two uses of the Kingdom of God in Jesus' teaching, there is an inevitable tension between the present and the future. In fact his vision of the Kingdom can only be understood if its present and future aspects are held in a creative tension. The future reign of God is assured, but — and here is where his own person embodies the good news — in the life, teaching, preaching and healing of Jesus, that reign of God is already being revealed. The Kingdom of God is seen in God's kingly activity breaking into history and human experience; and that activity is motivated towards the salvation of his people. He is now visiting and redeeming his people. That is Jesus' own message about his own ministry.

And how and where is the Kingdom of God being manifested? The answer is in the sphere of human, individual experience. It is in the changing of human lives that God's reign is supremely revealed, when man glimpses the vision of God and becomes fully alive, fully what he was created to be, if only in this life for an instant. 'The glory of God is a living man, and the life of man is the vision of God,' said Irenaeus, uttering a profound truth for all time. And as man stretches out the hand of faith, itself a gift, to appropriate the blessings of the Kingdom that are revealed before his very eyes — in healings, exorcisms, changed lives — so for a moment of glory he is caught up into the domain of God's kingly rule, glimpses the vision of God and experiences the glorious future in the eternal present. It is the Transfiguration experience, an experience that will in God's good time (*ho kairos*) recur, but for the moment must be left behind as the descent is made to the plain. The vision, however, can and must live on and, because Jesus has now risen from the dead and is alive for evermore, can and must be shared with everyone (Matt. 17.9). It is kept redolent through prayer: 'Thy Kingdom come . . . on earth as it is in heaven', a petition for the future consummation of that which has already begun in the believer's experience, with the sure hope that God will continue his kingly activity until it reaches its consummation at the end time and 'God is all in all'.

In his formative work *The Vision of God*,[3] Bishop Kenneth Kirk declared: 'Christianity had come into the world with a double purpose, to offer men the vision of God, and to call them to the pursuit of that vision.' I believe the order of that experience is important and reflects the biblical experience. Some scholars[4] now affirm that there is to be found in the Old Testament a proclamation of the salvific activity of God on behalf of his people, to which the Law is an accepting response. It is argued that after the entry into Canaan, a renewal festival used to be held at which was recited the history of God's saving acts on behalf of his people. This was followed by a recitation of the Commandments. In other words, they were presented with a vision of God by a proclamation of his saving acts. They then were faced with the decision as to whether they would accept this vision, this saving activity of God on their behalf. The affirmative response was to hear and accept the Commandments, the purpose of which was to extend and deepen their relationship with the God who had done such great things for their salvation. The carrying out of the Commandments made possible the experience of further salvific gifts God had to give the nation. The burden of emphasis in the Old Testament may therefore be rather on a gospel to which men respond by obedience to the Law, and not the other way round.

This process of vision and response was also capable of development according to changing circumstances and on-going experience. For instance, when the prophets reproached the people for not keeping the Law, in actual fact they were lamenting their lack of response to God's saving acts and their breaking of their relationship with the God who had done such great things to effect their salvation.

But when they proclaimed the judgement of God upon his people, they also held out the hope of new circum-stances which would open the way to a new saving activity of God which, in its turn, would result in a new response by the people. We therefore find both Jeremiah and Ezekiel foreseeing the chance of a new covenant made possible by a new initiative of God's saving activity. This new vision would lead to a new relationship, because the response of obedience to the Law would be that much easier as it would be part of their very being:

> 'The time is coming,' declares the Lord,
>   'when I will make a new covenant
> with the house of Israel
>   and with the house of Judah.
> It will not be like the covenant
>   I made with their forefathers
> when I took them by the hand
>   to lead them out of Egypt,
> because they broke my covenant,
>   though I was a husband to them,'
>   declares the Lord.
> 'This is the covenant that I will make
>   with the house of Israel
> after that time,' declares the Lord.

'I will put my law in their minds
    and write it on their hearts.
I will be their God,
    and they will be my people.
No longer will a man teach his
        neighbour,
    or a man his brother, saying, "Know
        the Lord,"
because they will all know me,
    from the least of them to the
        greatest,'
                declares the Lord.
'For I will forgive their wickedness
    and will remember their sins no more.'
                    (Jer. 31.31–4)

This new vision and new relationship form the burden of the New Testament message. In the person of Jesus Christ, God comes among us to effect this new relationship and offers a new vision to man that will guide his feet into the way of peace. The dominant centrepiece of this vision, as we have seen above, is the Kingdom of God, and Jesus is at pains to open people's eyes to it through the ordinary things of life — a seed, leaven, a wedding feast. Vision consists in seeing the extraordinary revealed in the ordinary. Jesus was constantly urging his disciples to be watchful, to have their eyes and ears open.

It was for the sake of this vision and as a response to it that Jesus made demands on the disciples. Having seen the vision, the response would be made in terms of putting one's hand to the plough, letting the dead bury their dead, being single-minded in following 'the Way', and taking up the cross daily. But all discipleship is consequent upon the seeing of the vision first and then seeking to express it in terms of daily life.

It was at the crisis points of life that Jesus offered people new vision, and especially through his healing ministry, which effected a double purpose. First, it was a demonstration of the breaking in of the Kingdom of God into this life, a manifestation of the future glory in the present reality. This was the way Jesus intended his miracles to be viewed, as signs of his Father's reign beginning to happen, signs of the healing of creation coming to pass. 'If I drive out demons by the Spirit of God, then the kingdom of God has come upon you' (Matt. 12.28).

Jesus' healing ministry also met people where they were, and not six feet above them or where it was considered they should be. This was borne in upon me during an interview on breakfast television, in which my friend Dr Peter Nixon and I were to face the bowling together. I knew that I had to take first ball and that it would be a fast one on the middle stump, something like 'Tell me, bishop, what do you mean by Christian healing?' Well, I had come armed with a few definitions, but mercifully Anne and I had prayed with a representative of Christian Communications in the lobby before going to make-up. Sure enough the first ball was pretty much word-for-word as envisaged, but as it was being bowled my mind was cleared of all those definitions and I heard myself saying (and so I claim no credit for it), 'Christian healing is Jesus Christ meeting you at the point of your need.' It was a precious gift that I shall always treasure. And of course it is just that: Jesus meeting people at the point of their need and therefore communicating with them and to them a totally new vision for their life. It is a true meeting of the divine with human need, of the Creator with the creature, of *the* Healer with the sick, of the One who alone can supply the needs of his people with those people in need. He meets them just where they are. He meets *us* just where we are. He meets *me* just where I am. And the meeting, because it is one of love, is not only journey's end as all lovers' meetings are, but also life's beginning, the new possibility of seeing visions and dreaming dreams. 'One thing I do know. I was blind but now I see' (John 9.25). The moment of the healing was the disclosure moment; for the writer of the fourth gospel, God's glory has been seen in his Son, and whoever has seen the Son has also seen the Father.

For St Paul the vision of God is also a reality. Using as a symbol the veil Moses put over his face to protect the Israelites from seeing the radiance of God reflected in his countenance, Paul declares that in Christ this veil is removed: 'Whenever anyone turns to the Lord, the veil is taken away.' His healing is also for a purpose: 'We, who with unveiled faces all reflect the Lord's glory, are being transformed into his likeness with ever-increasing glory, which comes from the Lord, who is the Spirit' (2 Cor. 3.16,18). The healing begins a process of total transformation. It is therefore never complete in itself. Rather it opens the person to a more constant vision of the Lord of glory, and that person is then able to reflect the glory on to others. That radiance is kept fresh by the response of discipleship in obedient acts, which make one 'apt' for the vision of God. And these acts are 'the acts of the whole person'. The vision is total and so also is the response, involving not only the whole person, but also the community: '*We* . . . all reflect . . . are being transformed.'[5]

The response of discipleship keeping a person apt for the vision of God is clearly seen in the book of Revelation. The seer was a tried disciple being punished for his unflinching witness to the truth of the gospel. He knew the Scriptures, and he knew obedience. He was also used to the regular worship and being 'in the Spirit on the Lord's Day'. In exile he kept this weekly tryst with his Lord and was immediately told to write (Rev. 1.10). What has happened is that the writer in his Sunday worship, alone in exile, has fallen under the hand of the Spirit who orders him to write a visionary meditation, and this he does obediently (the normal response to the vision in the natural order of things) 'through meditating into a new unity several old scriptures relevant to his purpose'.[6] The prophets of Israel had seen visions and recorded them in the written word; John pondered upon these written records 'until they fused into fresh shapes, expressive of a fuller truth'. Here we see the visions leading to a strengthening of John's discipleship when most needed; but we also see his discipleship making him ever more watchful and ready to receive new visions, culminating in the vision of the new Jerusalem and the voice from the throne proclaiming, 'I am making everything new!' (Rev. 21.5).

With this close overlapping of the vision and discipleship it is not surprising to find some of the doctors of the eastern Church expressing the view that the vision of God *is* discipleship. Gregory of Nyssa (*c* 330 – 95), brother to Basil of Caesarea, writing in his *Life of Moses* declares that the following of God with all one's heart and soul and powers is to see God. Elsewhere he writes that to 'imitate the divine nature' is consistently to follow the pattern of God's life as revealed in Jesus. Discipleship is a faithful following and living out of the vision of God.

Frank Wright underlines the primacy of vision in his brief but masterly work on *The Pastoral Nature of the Ministry*.[7] He quotes Simone Weil: 'the *looking* is what saves us', and

Ian Ramsey who also called attention to the primacy of vision and the necessity to see. Ramsey took A. N. Whitehead's description of religion as his starting point: 'Religion is the vision of something which stands beyond, behind, and within, the passing flux of immediate things, something which is real, and yet waiting to be realized . . .' When human experience takes on an extra dimension and depth, Ramsey argued, when a 'disclosure moment' is experienced, then that experience is religious.[8] It is at that point that vision comes, 'when the penny drops', or 'when I see'.

The person who is saved, made whole, is the person who responds to a vision of God's life in Christ. The task of the Church is therefore to open up moments of disclosure, occasions of vision where the people may truly see, 'when society can rediscover some sense of the sublime', in short, where the Kingdom of God can become a present reality. The responsibility for opening up such moments of vision and inspiration is laid upon those called to positions of leadership in the Church. And as Ramsey said, we only give a lead by displaying in our utterances or in other ways that which inspires us. The implication is that, if we don't feel inspired, it is best to keep silent, though every preacher knows that just at that moment when his or her feelings are those of emptiness and ineptitude, at that point, if those feelings are acknowledged, God is able to enter the situation and take over. The needful part for Christian leaders to play today is little different from any other age. It might well be summed up in one word: to contemplate. To contemplate the things of God, seeking to behold his way, his will, his involvement in the small things of life as well as the vastness of the universe; to allow the spaciousness and timelessness of the divine to enter through them the human arena; to create oases of stillness and vision through the things they have contemplated, and then *to hand on* those things they have contemplated. *Contemplare et contemplata tradere* — to contemplate and to hand on the things contemplated.

The true contemplative is a person on the move, who is going somewhere. He may be 'standing in the temple with God' (presumably the original meaning of con*templa*te), but the feeling emitted by his stance is that he is about to set out, he is a pilgrim on a journey of growth. He has been still in order to know his God a little more and so feels equipped to journey on to the next staging post. He is someone on the move who is being moved on, motivated by the Holy Spirit of movement. And because he has contemplated, he has *seen*, not necessarily with the outward eye, but more probably with the inner consciousness, the truth and the direction of his journey. With St Paul he is equipped with a vision of what lies ahead and is able to 'press on towards the goal to win the prize for which God has called me heavenwards in Christ Jesus' (Phil. 3.14).

The Christian leader has an obligation to put before men and women again in our time the significance of their destiny. He or she will only accomplish this if they are a person of vision, someone who has not only seen the Lord in mountain-top visions but sees him in the ordinary things of life, and can so illuminate life for others that the ordinary is transfigured into the extraordinary. The destiny we are all called to fulfil is the undertaking of that journey to wholeness that leads to maturity, 'until we all reach unity in the faith and in the knowledge of the Son of God and become mature, attaining to the whole measure of the fullness of Christ' (Eph. 4.13).

To attain this vision and keep it unsullied, Jesus himself had to pay the highest price, a cost that anyone must sit down and count who will follow the vision they are given. He could fulfil his destiny only at the price of loneliness, unpopularity, betrayal and eventually death on the cross, but it was for *the joy that was before him* that he endured; the joy that the Kingdom of heaven would be opened to all believers. His victory came through continuing on the journey. The Kingdom of God itself may well be a road, a direction, a movement, a vision. The only sure point is God, and him reigning, revealed by him who is 'The Way'.

5

People of the Way

A doctor has well-trained eyes. He has been trained to perceive the true state of a person's health from a searching look into their eyes. It is fortunate that a doctor wrote the first history of the early Church.

Luke the beloved physician lived up to his profession's known acumen in the sphere of perception. He began by examining the evidence, all available witnesses, and the oral traditions that he found among the early Christians (Luke 1. 1–4). But more was to come. He must have kept on asking himself, 'Where are these Christians going? What is the purpose of their journey? What are they trying to say to the world? Are they being faithful to their Master's vision?' His clinical mind was an asset for the work he set himself to do and has left us with a rich legacy in his two volumes. It is the second, the book of the Acts of the Apostles, in which he tries to answer these insistent questions as he ponders on and records the history of the life and times of the apostles.

I like to imagine him sitting down to write volume two, gazing into space to see visions and to discern where he is being led. He obviously has a vivid awareness of the leading of the Holy Spirit. He has been part of the story himself, accompanying St Paul as his personal physician on some of his missionary journeys. Is there a purpose, a theme, a key to all of these experiences?

I believe his professional eye saw a movement onward and outward 'into all the world' (under the guidance of the

Spirit of Movement). It was rather like the ripples on a pond after you have thrown a stone into the middle. The concentric circles increase in number and size until the whole pond is engulfed in the movement of the water. That was what was happening in the world as the message of Christianity was handed on, and still continues today. Jesus Christ has come into the centre of our existence, into the midst of the world's life. His presence and power are facts that are now being proclaimed, and the 'movement' is gradually traversing the whole world. The journeys of these early Christians, filled with the life and message of the world's Saviour, Luke discerned as the cause of these powerful vibrations in ever-increasing circles that were moving onward and outward. 'You will receive power when the Holy Spirit comes on you; and you will be my witnesses in Jerusalem, and in all Judaea and Samaria, and to the ends of the earth' (Acts 1.8). There, in essence, is a summary of Luke's story, which he records as the final words of Jesus before his ascension.

He closed his book when the gospel reached Rome, but 'the ends of the earth' as far as the Roman Empire was concerned (and any Roman legionary of the day would have told you without hesitation) was Britain. There are many who believe that St Paul came to Britain, between his imprisonments in Rome. Certainly there was a Christian cell at this 'end of the earth' shortly after Pentecost, probably through the journeyings of Joseph of Arimathea, whose name is linked with Glastonbury. Be that as it may, Luke saw the purpose of the Christian enterprise as a journey of witness until the whole was 'leavened', just like Jesus' parable of the Kingdom. It was essential for the operation that those taking part should move onward and outward. No wonder St Paul was his hero.

If this was the scale and scheme of his purpose in writing, the next question facing the good doctor was what he should record out of all the available material. What were the important facts that he wanted his readers to take to their hearts? He obviously had to connect up the narrative with his previous volume, the Gospel that bears his name. He therefore re-told the story of Jesus' ascension, which he dated forty days after Easter day, a dating the Church has followed in its calendar. The next event was the coming of the Holy Spirit, which as it was on the feast of Pentecost, must be fifty days after Easter. There were the two important historical events of immense consequence that Luke recorded as the overture to his 'opus'. What next?

Every writer has his own idiosyncracies (don't you know it, patient reader!) and mercifully, to assist us in answering this next question concerning what Luke wanted to ensure did not escape the notice of our dull wits, he left us a clue. As the bellman in Lewis Carroll's *Hunting of the Snark* declared as he angrily tolled his bell: 'What I tell you three times is true', so Luke repeats important events or speeches two or three times when he considers them to be of heightened significance. He therefore records the conversion of St Paul, one of the most significant events in Christian history, no less than three times (Acts 9, 22 and 26); while 'the Gentile Pentecost' in the house of Cornelius, an event hardly less significant since it changed the ethos of the primitive Christian community from a Jewish sect to a worldwide religious movement, he records twice (Acts 10 and 11).

The other event for which he takes a full canvas immediately follows the opening chapters that describe the ascension and Pentecost. In this case the repetition occurs within the one narrative: Peter delivers two homilies on the subject of the story — the healing of the crippled man at the Temple gate called Beautiful. Luke takes two whole chapters (3 and 4) to tell the story.

Jesus had probably passed this man time and again as he entered the Temple. Why didn't he stop to heal him? The New Testament word for time, you will recall, means opportunity or the right time, God's time. Perhaps there is a right time on our journey to wholeness for us to receive physical healing or inner healing, a time that God has ordained for this to happen, when it can give *Him* the greater glory. Here was the right time, the God-given opportunity for this cripple to receive healing, when his healing could contribute to the dissemination of the gospel message as crowds flocked to the Temple. Peter's intuitive wisdom caused him to stop at that particular time on that particular day, and he gave the man all that he asked for — and more: 'Silver and gold I do not have, but what I have I give you. In the name of Jesus Christ of Nazareth, walk' (Acts 3.6). Not only was he able to walk, but he walked in the name of Jesus Christ. And here, it seems to me, is encapsulated the whole truth about Christian healing. So many who desire healing have never thought further than the physical. Now I admit that when illness strikes it is very hard to think of anything else than the sheer physical suffering. It is natural that this takes over our whole world and we long to be free of this imprisonment and pain. Jesus, in his compassion for such people and in the way he healed them, showed that it was wholly right for them to seek physical healing. But in every case he also showed them a deeper dimension to life. He lifted their spirit also and changed their life by giving it new hope and turning it God's way. He demonstrated that there is a deeper healing we also need; in addition to having our symptoms cured, *the true end of healing is being freed to walk on our journey to wholeness in the company of Jesus Christ.* Healing by itself will help us surmount many obstacles in this life. Christian healing is the healing Christ wills to give us in order to equip us not only for a deeper experience of the joys of this life, but also for that which is to come. The journey to wholeness has this double dimension. Little wonder the man not only 'jumped to his feet and began to walk,' but also went with them into the Temple 'walking and jumping *and praising God'* (Acts 3.8). If , as C. S. Lewis said, praise is inner health made audible, the cripple obviously made everyone aware that he had been physically and spiritually healed.

When a crowd assembled, Peter used the 'opportunity' to proclaim the gospel message: 'It is Jesus' name and the faith that comes through him that has given this *complete healing* to him, as you can all see' (Acts 3.16). It is important that we are not distracted from the true path of our journey into a byway to incomplete healing. The main road of the journey is to complete wholeness, which means far more than the relief of physical symptoms. It is nothing less than a walk with Christ.

Peter and John were of course arrested for their pains, but that gave them a chance to witness once again on the following day, and this time to the whole Sanhedrin, which Peter did with refreshing directness as befits the proclamation of the gospel. Warnings for him to stop his witness were in vain, and it is interesting that the continuous praising of God by the people for what had happened led to the defeat of the opposition upon whom fell an unaccustomed indecisiveness about how to punish them.

Before we draw any conclusions from this remarkable story to which Luke gave such prominence, let us observe its ending. Peter and John returned to the house of their fellow Christians, who presumably had been at prayer for them since their arrest. After a great welcome they fell to prayer again, first of praise and thanksgiving, followed by a significant petition: 'Lord consider their threats and enable your servants to speak your word with great boldness. Stretch out your hand to heal and perform miraculous signs and wonders through the name of your holy servant Jesus' (Acts 4.29 – 30). It is important for a church in mission to take to heart the three parts of this petition. First there is a surrender of all opposition and problems to the Lord. The verb used here for 'consider' is a Greek word used of the gods looking upon and overseeing human affairs. Here it is a prayer for God to take charge of those who oppose his word. Petitioners surrender this problem, which will loom large in each generation, into the Lord's hands, and *leave it* with him. We must learn from them to do the same.

In the second place they ask for one quality alone to help them co-operate with the enabling power of the Holy Spirit in their preaching of the gospel: that is, boldness. They could have asked for anything; but in the face of opposition they asked for boldness. That has not always been the prime quality in the proclamation of the gospel. It is, however, the one quality necessary in the task we have been set of witnessing on our journey to the saving and healing power of God. If the gospel has no cutting edge in our generation, it is because of our lack of boldness. We have accommodated our gospel to the ethos of the world more frequently than we have confronted the world with the cutting edge of the gospel. There must be a possibility open to faith, otherwise the world has no purpose beyond its own existence. The time is late for such a change; boldness on the part of Christians is an urgent priority for prayer.

The third part of the prayer follows on in natural

progression from the first two parts. If the opposition and problems are fully surrendered to the Lord, if he has bold servants to be the channels of his work here on earth, then we shall be witnesses of his power to heal as his hand is still stretched out to put his Father's world to rights. The signs and wonders inevitably follow a fearless proclamation of the good news of Jesus Christ.

This is pretty heady stuff, but the place was shaken after their prayer, which was immediately answered. They received the blessing of the Holy Spirit, who moved them on in their journey by giving them the very boldness in the proclamation for which they had prayed.

Let us now turn to the reasons for Luke's long and detailed treatment of this episode. Why does he give such a simple story such pride of place and such space in his history? As a doctor, he would take especial note of the methodology used by the apostles in the furtherance of their mission. He would observe that they were closely faithful to Jesus' commission to proclaim his good news both by preaching and healing. Their practice would make it plain to Luke that this was invariably a 'both/and' and never an 'either/or' alternative. The two strands of proclamation always went in parallel. This methodology so impressed him by its obviously effective communication of the message, that he became determined to hand on this method to successive generations of Christians. It was in fact Jesus' own method, and to practise it was an act of obedience to the direct command of Jesus to proclaim the gospel in this way. Luke was therefore underlining in bold colours the obedience of the early Church to its Lord's commission. In effect he was saying, 'This is the way: walk in it. This is part of the Church's own journey to wholeness.' Times of dis-ease in the Church have usually coincided with an unfaithfulness or lack of obedience to the Lord's bidding and commission. The search again in our time to be obedient in regard to the preach/heal commission, should augur well for a new springtime for the Church, despite some appearances to the contrary. It is a happy memory that Pope John XXIII invited the bishops of the Roman Catholic Church to study these early chapters of Acts as an act of preparation for their conclave, Vatican II. Many believe that his prayerful initiative has led to a springtime in all the Churches. 'The prayer of a righteous man is powerful and effective' (James 5.16).

Another significant point which Luke discerned from his observance of the life of the early Church was the name Christians gave to themselves. Before they were called 'Christ's men' or Christians in Antioch, they called themselves 'people of the Way'. Saul was sent to Damascus 'so that if he found any there who belonged to the Way, whether men or women, he might take them as prisoners to Jerusalem' (Acts 9.2). Apollos 'was a learned man with a thorough knowledge of the Scriptures' and 'he had been instructed in the Way of the Lord.' However, though he spoke out boldly from a deep knowledge of the Old Testament and indeed 'taught about Jesus accurately', 'he knew only the baptism of John'. For this reason Priscilla and Aquila 'invited him to their own home and explained to him the Way of God more adequately' (Acts 18. 24—6).

The name of 'the Way' was therefore still current in Ephesus, some time after the name of 'Christian' had been given to the disciples at Antioch. Indeed, three months after Paul's arrival there on his third missionary journey, opposition to 'the Way' caused him to transfer his base of operations from the synagogue to the lecture hall of Tyrannus. Worse was to come. 'Disturbance about the

71

Way', fomented by Demetrius and his fellow silversmiths, caused the total uproar in the city that led to the riot in the theatre and the frenzied shouting of the crowd, 'Great is Artemis of the Ephesians' (Acts 19.9 and 23–41).

It is also interesting that Felix, who examined Paul after his arrest, had taken the trouble to make himself well-informed about 'the Way'. It was a movement that those in authority took seriously. Those who followed Christ were seen to be a community on the move, a people with a purpose. They proclaimed Jesus as Lord for all peoples, as 'the Way' for the world.

The final proof to the early Church of the cosmic implications of the gospel message was the Cornelius episode in Acts 10. This event was a watershed in the history of the Church since it convinced the leadership that their thinking, which at first went no further than the Church being little more than a Jewish sect, was far too narrow. The Christian Church was indeed for all peoples. There was no-one, indeed no-thing, for whom Christ had not died and risen again.

Luke frequently and significantly records a healing at the time of a widening of the Church's consciousness. As we are learning again in our time, these signs are not only for the benefit of those healed; rather they enlarge the spiritual perception of the whole healing community, especially of those through whom the healing Christ worked to effect the sign. Two healings prefaced the Cornelius episode itself, those of Aeneas and Tabitha or Dorcas. Perhaps they were meant to prepare Peter for the 'Gentile Pentecost' in the house of Cornelius. At any rate they were a sign of the imminent extension of the Church's boundaries (Acts 9.32–43). There are also further illustrations of this in Acts, for example the healing of the cripple in Lystra,

(Acts 14.8–10), which led to the demythologizing of the Greek gods and further Christian teaching, prior to Paul's own healing after being stoned, and the further missionary expansion in Derbe. Again, the healing of the fortune-telling slave girl in Philippi (Acts 16.16–18) led first to Paul's and Silas' imprisonment but then to the conversion of the jailer and his household, presumably the prisoners also, and a healthy confrontation with the unjust custodians of the law the next day. But it also happened that the whole event formed the prelude of Paul's missionary work not only in Greece but in Europe. The healing Christ was leading his Church in his Way, holding out an ever greater wholeness if his servants would move onwards and outwards at his bidding. A healing seemed to take on a new significance as a signal for that move forward.

Further stages of development can be discerned in the New Testament. By the time of the Corinthian letters (which were probably written before Luke/Acts), Paul tries to formulate the gifts of the Spirit among which he mentions 'gifts of healing' (1 Corinthians 12.9) as well as 'miraculous powers' and later in the same chapter, 'workers of miracles' are listed as a fourth order in the Church, followed by 'those having gifts of healing'. The Corinthians were misusing these gifts because they were employing them for selfish ends, in fact to self-glorification. Love was absent. They had failed to remember that God was the Giver and the Church as a whole the recipient. The gifts were given to the whole Body and for the purpose of mutual service. The gifts of healing and miraculous powers can never be ends in themselves; they have a wider purpose. They are given for the building up of the Body of Christ and the extension of God's Kingdom. And the greatest of them is love (1 Corinthians 13).

A later development still is found in the letter of James. The gifts of healing seem to have become part of the normal ministry of the church as exercised by the elders. The sick person is taught to 'call the elders of the church' who will 'pray over him and anoint him with oil in the name of the Lord' (James 5.14). Presumably the 'praying over' is done with the laying on of hands which is part of the sacrament of anointing. The writer goes on to say that 'the prayer offered in faith will make the sick person well; the Lord will raise him up. If he has sinned, he will be forgiven.' The prayers of faith and forgiveness are obviously elements of a healing ministry and one would still be inclined to call them 'gifts'. Certainly, as the ministers of Christ's Church go faithfully about their ministry, particularly when caring for God's poor which includes the sick, they are creating disclosure situations for God's gifts to be given, for the benefit of the whole Church and for the glory of God. The signs that follow herald a move forward by the people of 'the Way', and the Christian community is advanced and enlarged as more and more turn to follow him who is the Way.

It is left to the apocalyptic writings of the visionary exile on the isle of Patmos to see the ultimate in the healing mission of God's people of the Way. The leaves on the trees, which are irrigated by the water flowing down the *middle walk-way* of the city, are for the healing of the nations. We must return to this vision in the final chapter.

6

The People of the Way Move On

Creation is ever expanding and constantly moving. It is subject to constant change as the evolutionary process inexorably moves on its way. That much science has shown us. It should not cause us surprise that the Creator God makes a three-fold response to that creation: by accepting it as it is, which includes an acceptance of each of us as we are; by providing us with the encouragement and ability to change, in conquering death and sin and by revealing that death leads to new life; and by the gift of the Spirit, who moved on the face of the waters and is the dynamic of change within us, that now moves us on and forms us into the being we are capable of becoming.

Movement is therefore a characteristic both of the Creator and of creation, a motive power towards immersion in life, to changing and being changed. Those who have known the 'hand' of God upon them are being moved on because they are servants of the Kingdom of God which itself is a dynamic concept. It is the very nature of the people of God to be on the move, to respond to the divine call to be on the way. And, as happens in all molecular and cell movements, the result is a community, a joining together for the next step in the process. 'All life is meeting and all true life is lived in community.' The evolution of the ecclesial community is so to lose its life in the whole that the whole is changed to the glory of God.

It is essential therefore that there is constant movement within the ecclesial community, to give these messages of change to the total world community, as well as ensuring that the life dynamic process goes on within the People of God and keeps them on their journey. *Veni Creator Spiritus* must be the constant prayer of the Church. In fact, though outward appearances may point to the contrary, there have been many such movements pointing the way to life and change within the last century or so, all of which have a message for the whole world community.

It was the Evangelical revival of the last century that brought about a Christian involvement in national politics and led, among other things, to the abolition of slavery. The Oxford Movement is dated from John Keble's Assize sermon which awoke not only a university but the whole nation, and particularly the inhabitants of its parsonage houses, where the *Tracts for the Times* were distributed, to new responsibilities and brought life and colour again to the nation's churches. The Ecumenical movement is usually dated from the Edinburgh conference in 1910 where the youthful William Temple was a steward. Few movements have had such a far-reaching effect on all the churches of Christendom and melted in two generations the frozen attitude in Christian relationships. Little wonder, with such pioneers as Temple and George Bell.

It may be of some significance that another movement began to stir at about the same time. I have told the story elsewhere,[1] but I want to underline some of the dates, facts and personalities. In 1905 James Moore Hickson, to whom the healing movement if we may call it such, owes much of its inspiration on a world scale, founded the Guild of Emmanuel (note the name), which was later to become the Divine Healing Mission. The Guild was to be a call to prayer, a call to Christian men and women to turn again to the healing Christ in giving themselves to prayer on behalf of the sick and needy. From the very beginning the healing movement has stood for a recalling of the Church to deep prayer. I believe that that initial emphasis on prayer is bearing fruit in this generation.

James Moore Hickson owed much to his mother's sensitive training. From the time he was fourteen she noticed that he seemed to have a gift of healing through touch. She began to pray with him that God would give him discernment and direction on the journey of life, as to how he wanted this gift to be used. The prayer of mother and son was answered beyond all doubt. Prayer was always the seed-bed of the healing dimension of the Church's ministry.

It is also to be noted that he was a layman. The laity of the churches have constantly led the way forward in the healing ministry. They have been people of prayer and some, like Dorothy Kerin, have been raised up by God, in her case literally from a bed of mortal sickness, to recall the Church in their time to the healing dimension of its ministry. The Church of Christ the Healer at Burrswood stands as a reminder to the people of God that prayer and praise to the Christ who heals is the *sine qua non* of this whole movement and ministry. That was the way Dorothy Kerin and James Moore Hickson led their fellow members of the people of God on the journey to wholeness. How very many they inspired to set out on that road! A new generation of people on the Way.

James Moore Hickson also visited the Archbishop of Canterbury in the same year. Randall Davidson responded to the inspiration of this young man by sending him out with the prophetic words: 'You go forth as the patrol of an army; I will lead the main body forward.' It has been a torch handed on to successive leaders in the Anglican Church, and the Church's healing ministry has been given a place at each Lambeth Conference during this century.[2]

One final point about this remarkable pioneer, James Moore Hickson. In that same year when he was only twenty years of age, he prophesied that Christ would again give his healing charisms to his Church in this century, and for two reasons: first, for the healing of the churches themselves, and second, to prepare them for the Second Coming. The healing of the churches is a primary factor in this whole movement and indeed in the healing of all ills. I shall never forget the challenge of a lay person who, at the end of a long letter, pleaded: 'Heal the Church and we shall all get well.' It was reminiscent of God's call to total obedience from his people after the Exodus and the promise of 'none of these diseases'. While there is any imbalance or distress in the human body, it is hard for that body to be entirely well. So also for the Body of Christ. The great hope held out to us is that while we are engaging in healing work, acting in obedience to the healing Christ and offering even the cup of cold water, a healing is coming to us as more and more we become one in *him*: 'that all of them may be one, Father, just as you are in me and I am in you. May they also be in us so that the world may believe that you have sent me' (John 17.21). The healing of his Body the Church is a continuing priority in Christ's high priestly intercession, for it is a necessary preliminary to his coming again.

The architect of the Life and Liberty movement also made a significant contribution to the healing movement. Possibly the one naturally flowed into the other. William Temple, the People's Archbishop, did not miss the significance of Jesus' very own ministry which met people at the point of their need. He had not been Bishop of Manchester long when a report of a working party set up by the 1920 Lambeth Conference was published in 1924. It produced a recommendation which in the main asked for three things. I somewhat frivolously call it the TCP formula, which at least has a healing sound!

1. Teaching on the whole Church's healing ministry.
2. Co-operation between doctors and clergy.
3. Prayer: the formation of intercessory prayer groups in every parish.

It is a good thing to pause for a moment to take in the fact that the Anglican leadership requested this action from the whole Anglican Communion as early as 1924. I believe it had a hitherto unnoticed, but nevertheless profound, effect upon William Temple. By the time of the next Lambeth Conference in 1930, at which this report was presented, Temple had been translated to York and in his new capacity was chosen as the preacher at the Conference's opening service in St. Paul's, Randall Davidson, who was to have preached, having died a few months before. His theme was the Majesty and Reign of God. The ending was one of many purple passages:

> While we deliberate, He reigns; when we decide wisely, He reigns; when we decide foolishly, He reigns; when we serve in humble loyalty, He reigns; when we serve him self-assertively, He reigns; when we rebel and seek to withold our service, He reigns — the Alpha and the Omega, which is, and which was, and which is to come, the Almighty.

It is not too far-fetched to assume that he had made a study of the theology upon which the teaching concerning the healing ministry should be based in response to the first suggestion of the 1924 report. He would know that the foundations of such teaching lie in the so-called Kingdom theology. God wills to reign in every part of his creation. Jesus came to proclaim that reign of his heavenly Father which was embodied in his own ministry and message. His preaching and his healing were all of a piece and formed the method by which the Kingdom was proclaimed. He commissioned his disciples to proclaim the same message, using the same method. Luke, as we have seen, shows how faithfully and obediently the apostles carried out their commission. Temple showed his adherence to such a gospel by the subject matter of his sermon to the 1930 Conference. He was, however, to prove himself totally faithful to his Master's example; by his action as well as by his word.

In 1942 he was translated to Canterbury from York. The English Church was to be deprived of one of its greatest leaders ever by his untimely death two years later. A few months before he died, he took an initiative which led to the formation of what is now the Churches' Council for Health and Healing. The significant fact is that the basic work it was given to do was to implement the TCP formula. This initiative, like all Temple's thought, was forty years ahead of its time.

But his wisdom and prophetic insight saw to it that the 'movement' not only possessed motivation, but also direction and a heart. Such was one of the greatest of William Temple's legacies which has hitherto remained unsung. His prophetic mind was able to discern that there would be a time beyond the present one of preoccupation with scientific analysis and proof. It would be a time when man would see the universe in its wholeness once more and experience the power of the God who created it and raised up Jesus again to redeem it. It would therefore be a time when man need no longer rationalize away the whole fiduciary framework upon which he based his belief and from which he was led to hope in an 'author and giver of life' beyond himself. It would be a time which might well be called a new age of the person. At a time when human life counted for far less than its worth, Temple felt acutely that people mattered. He was not called the People's Archbishop for nothing. His was a Saviour who met people at the point of their need, in short, the Christ who heals in order to proclaim his Father's reign. And, as he showed in *Christus Veritas*, the healing given by Christ was a deep and inner healing which led to the dethroning of the self in man and the enthroning of Christ, the true man, the centre of all existence. 'The self is capable of complete satisfaction (? wholeness) in proportion as it is left outside the field of its own attention.' To this Temple added a footnote: 'In other words, joy is the fruit of humility.' That says more about true healing than much of what has been written on the subject. After all, humility was the virtue that Christ the Healer made his own.

Had Temple lived on after the war,[3] his theological insights about the Kingdom might have been developed into a new work and so encouraged academic theologians to move forward on another journey. That was not to be. Instead, few seemed able to interpret the reign of God to a post-war generation greatly longing for a message of hope, and so all remained depressed under the nuclear mushroom cloud that was to overhang several generations with a pall of gloom. As I have said before, possibly it will be the physicists who will supply the breakthrough of fresh hope by teaching a new world generation of the wholeness of the universe in which it resides. It will be somewhat ironical if it is the new scientists who will provide the fiduciary framework in whose paramaters a new generation of theologians will be able to lead the people of God on a forward journey of discovery.

If the teaching is still in a stage of development, what about the co-operation between doctors and clergy? Are the healing professions any more healed together? I suspect this rapprochement is also waiting for the new fiduciary framework, but already there are signs that a new pattern of relationships between the healing professions is gradually emerging. This is in itself a sign of hope that the new framework of faith is beginning to be laid.

For some time there has been widespread dissatisfaction, not least in the profession, with the present medical model, which views man as a machine, a system of physical processes, which remains passive — 'patient' — while the experts use their skills to negate disease in the body and improve its health. There has also been a similar disenchantment in the churches with a 'spiritual' view of life that concerns itself with the treatment of the soul alone, in isolation from the body in which it is rooted. Both views isolate God from some part of life, which is no longer a whole but a composition of fragments. Contemporary Christians, however, are regaining a vision of God in our time as the One in whom the principle of wholeness has its origin and fulfilment. He is indeed the Alpha and the Omega, the Lord of all life in its totality. A new people of the Way is on the move.

With the re-emergence of the idea of wholeness in Christianity, rooted in the Godhead itself, and with the re-emergence in science of a wholistic view of the universe, perhaps the foundations of this new fiduciary framework are already being laid. This is significant for the coming together of medicine and Christianity, especially when applied to the concept of health. For the term 'wholeness' becomes increasingly meaningful for both since it is descriptive not only of the unity of the personality, but also of the healing process itself. It is this concept of wholeness that holds out the greatest hope for the coming together of the healing professions. And even though not all in medicine will acknowledge the contribution that Christianity has to make, the vast majority would acknowledge that a sense of purpose or a meaningful orientation is necessary to the wholeness of a person, indeed to life itself. Christians would think of this as the spiritual factor and would see spiritual therapy as the vital contribution they would be able to offer. The most health-giving, wholistic and meaningful orientation that can be offered in the Christian view is a relationship with God, the source of all wholeness. That relationship is incarnated in the person of Jesus Christ, and Christians see him as the norm for what it means to be whole as well as the source of wholeness in the lives of those who accept him as Lord, Saviour and Healer. It is this kind of 'other' relationship to which Carl Jung referred when he stated 'among all my patients in the second half of life, there has not been one whose problem in the last resort was not that of finding a religious outlook on life'. The person who has another dimension to their life, in particular that relationship with the Christ who heals, has a head start on the journey to wholeness. The fact that this is gaining acceptance in medical circles may well provide the framework within which can be constructed a new partnership between the Church and Medicine in the caring for people with which both are entrusted.

There are encouraging signs that a new climate of co-operation is emerging. At the very least there seems to be a desire for dialogue at every level. The media coverage of some of the major ethical questions being faced in medicine today ensures a wide level of discussion. I hope it assures doctors that they don't and won't have to face such major issues alone. At another level, the rebuilding of a clinic for a general practice and of an adjacent Baptist church in a town centre, which came about simultaneously, provided the opportunity for fruitful dialogue and planning concerning future co-operation.

Exciting moves are in fact taking place. The Churches' Council for Health and Healing, under the present director, a Roman Catholic layman, now has a specifically medical department after its merger with the old Institute of Religion and Medicine. The Council has had a working party with the Royal College of Practitioners and produced a useful report on whole person medicine. It has its offices in the crypt of St Marylebone Parish Church alongside a doctor's surgery and other therapy and counselling rooms. It is a 'sign' of the working together of church and medicine, appropriately in a very 'medical' area, adjacent to Wimpole Street and Harley Street. It is an exercise in the city to promote this working together, just as Burrswood, near Tunbridge Wells, is a concentrated 'sign' of the integration of this work in a country setting, with the benefit of not only the Church of Christ the Healer, but of a nursing home with thirty-one beds and superb grounds.[4]

I think we ought at this point to recognize the contributions made by psychiatry to the dialogue between religion and medicine. Somewhat like Poland, which has been called the football of Europe, psychiatry has also been kicked around both by Medicine and the Church. In point of fact it has done much to bring them once more together. As Dr David Enoch has pointed out in his book *Healing the Hurt Mind*,[5] the Christian faith and clinical psychiatry reinforce the tenets of each other. In both is to be found a respect for man. A Christian says it all when he declares his

84

belief that God became man. The first President of the Royal Society of Psychiatrists, Sir Martin Roth, once said, 'Man is always more than he knows about himself and perhaps always will be.' Again, both lay emphasis on the wholeness of man, especially the closeness between the physical, the psychological and the spiritual. Both look on man as having a flaw — 'All have sinned and come short of the glory of God' — but both proclaim that man can change and be victorious. Whether drugs or psychotherapy are used, or Christian prayer and sacrament, both reach out to man in persuasion and love. In fact they both tackle one of man's greatest burdens — guilt. Of course, guilt may be pathological and therefore disappear when illness is cured. But it may be theological, a sin against God, needing spiritual treatment. As Dr Enoch says, nothing will clear this kind of guilt apart from the accepted forgiveness of Christ. At times there also needs to be a forgiveness of oneself.

More than anything they come together in their mutual emphasis on the importance of love in the life of man. Psychiatry declares that love and empathy are essential in the relationship with a patient. A Christian looks to his God and sees his love to be so great that he sent his own Son who by his life, death and resurrection not only taught us to love but also empowered us to do so.

I have emphasized only the positive factors, and of course there are factors on the other side. But it seems to me that this coming together by Christianity and psychiatry and finding so much common ground, has given the whole Religion-Medicine dialogue a shot in the arm and affirmed what is noblest in both in their care of man in distress or disease. The basic element of the future healing community must surely be a healed partnership and harmonious working together of the healing professions.

It seems that the concept of the healing community may

be a sign for our time, our particular juncture on the journey to wholeness. What is the essence of such a community? The New Testament views fellowship (*koinonia*) first and foremost in relationship to God, to the Father through or with the Son in union with the Holy Spirit. 'God, who has called you into fellowship with his Son Jesus Christ our Lord . . .' (1 Cor. 1.9). 'May the grace of the Lord Jesus Christ, and the love of God, and the fellowship of the Holy Spirit be with you all' (2 Cor. 13.14). Indeed it seems hard to envisage any community that is going to care for and satisfy the deep needs of its members without a strong Godward orientation. Only an awareness of the Creator God gives a fuller awareness of the needs of his creation. I believe this needs saying. In a pluralist society I also believe this is the only way to begin to lay the foundations of a healing community, for all religions and cultures have this point in common — an awareness of the divine and of their oneness with creation.

In the New Testament writings of the apostolic period we find a significant emphasis on the fact of God being the source of unity of human kind. 'There is one God, and the unity of the human race is rooted and grounded in the being of God. It is from divine unity that human unity derives. The idea of human unity is a central one in early Christianity.'[6] The theme of this new creation is contained in the letter to the Galatians, where Paul asserts that we enjoy this unity with God and therefore with each other 'through faith in Christ Jesus, for all of you who were baptized into Christ have clothed yourselves with Christ. There is neither Jew nor Greek, slave nor free, male nor female, for you are all one in Christ Jesus' (Gal. 3.26–8). In the final chapter (Gal. 6.15) he summarizes his theme: 'Neither circumcision nor uncircumcision means anything;

86

what counts is a new creation.' This is further developed
and brought to a conclusion in the letter to the Ephesians,
where 'the theme of human unity, and indeed of the entire
creation, is placed in a theological framework'.[7] God's plan
was 'to be put into effect when the times will have reached
their fulfilment — to bring all things in heaven and on earth
together under one head, even Christ' (Eph. 1.10). The
created order was destined to be a unity in God through the
work of Christ. 'Now in Christ Jesus you who once were far
away have been brought near through the blood of Christ'
(Eph. 2.13). In fact the whole letter views life, and the
Christian life in particular, as a sign of what true life should
be, as a movement towards a fulfilled and mature life in the
world community, a life 'hid with Christ in God' who gives
order and unity to the whole.

It is for this reason that Christians must continually be on
the move to create signs of this new creation, signs of hope
in a world without hope, signs of community in a disrupted
world, signs of healing where there is disease, distress and
disunity. The early Christians were quick to realize the
needs of their time. In a world that had gone away from
God, they knew they had to live a sign of God's presence.
The Holy Spirit of movement, unity and truth, led them, as
we read in those early chapters in Acts, to be such a sign in a
disbelieving world, such a light in the darkness of violent
disbelief. We read how 'they devoted themselves to the
apostles' teaching and to the fellowship, to the breaking of
bread and to prayer' (Acts 2.42). I have always felt this to be
one of the most important words given to us from Scripture.
Here was the framework for the lifestyle of the Christian
community, whose destiny was to be a sign of the unity of
all creation. Every part of it spoke of a relationship with God
through Christ in the power of the Spirit, lived out in the

service of humanity until God was all in all. The teaching, fellowship, breaking of bread, prayer – all pointed Godward and drew the believer into a relationship with Christ in God in order to fulfil his essential destiny as a living part of creation, to be fully human and fully alive.

It is this community into which we are called, and which we are called to live, work and die for, in every generation. The answering of the call with our 'Amen' (Yes, Lord, I am willing to set out) is a profound 'Yes' to our call to *be* a living part of creation. And in Christ there is the possibility of being that new creation (2 Cor. 5.17) *together*, reconciled, ransomed, healed, restored, forgiven, in the community of all creation, of which the Christian cells are but signs, but vital signs and pointers to all people on the way. The ultimate is God's Kingdom; the destination is a healed creation, over which in 'timeless potency' the Holy Spirit continues to brood. In the meantime we travel as the People of the Way, the divine community on the move, the dynamic fellowship of the Holy Spirit, the Body of Christ; and always we are empowered to move *forward* to the glory of God the Father.

7

Journey's end is Lovers' meeting

When Jesus taught his disciples to pray he gave them large themes. He prescribed a vast canvas for their prayer. They were to pray as part of the world-wide family, their eyes lifted to heaven (Our Father in heaven). The first request was for a hallowing of the Father's name, and because for a Jew the name signified the total personality, this meant the worship of God on a cosmic scale (on earth, as in heaven). The second request was made for the coming of the Kingdom, a supplication that God would reign in every part of his creation, not only in the billions of cells that go to form my own being but in the whole universe with which I am totally interconnected and conjoined. This is a prayer for the healing of all creation. The third request was for the Father's will to be done, again on a cosmic scale, not only by mankind but also by the 'principalities and powers'. The opening sections of the Lord's Prayer are utterly breathtaking. We are praying for nothing less than the transfiguration of the world, indeed of the universe, according to the will and through the power of God.

> Thou art coming to a King:
> Great petitions with thee bring.

This wider dimension of prayer must never be lost under a welter of personal requests, however important they may seem to be.

It will be noticed that the whole prayer is prayed

corporately, since the first person plural is used throughout. We pray together as People of the Way. And in the personal petitions which follow the universal, we first recall the fact that God has always been the provider of food for the Way throughout the pilgrimage of his People. We therefore ask as part of the journeying People for the daily bread. There is a hint here that not only the material bread is meant, but also the spiritual and mental nourishment which we need to equip us for the Way. The canvas of the prayer constantly seems to have a wider dimension than readily meets the eye.

The next petition is a request for the obtaining of that kind of relationship without which it would be impossible to survive as a People on the Way – mutual forgiveness. We need God's forgiveness to become his pilgrim people; we also need to forgive others, and indeed to allow them to forgive us. We also need to forgive ourselves. This kind of forgiveness is the only basis for life that has to move on. It is the only commodity that will ensure healthy relationships for God's people as they travel. It is easy to see how the lack of it disrupts life – in broken families, warring nations, and in much of the sickness we see around us. The lack of forgiveness, shown in angry resentment, overtly or inwardly, is responsible for much of the dis-ease in society, both individual and corporate. The lengths to which Christ went on the cross in order to procure the forgiveness of our sins and those of the whole world should rivet the importance of this petition deep into our consciousness. 'The benefit of absolution' is the constant and crying need of the world in which we are pilgrims and of which for a span we are part.

The final petition I take to be for guidance, an avoidance of being tested above the threshold we are able to bear and

90

a deliverance from the powers of darkness should we stray beyond that point. How very many pitfalls should we have avoided had we only paused and waited, to pray for guidance and listen to the prompting of the Lord. And if this is the experience of God's People of the Way, what about those who are hell-bent (*sic*) on going in the opposite direction to God's way? Once again, it can only underline the gravity of this petition, the need for God's people to seek guidance for the Way at every step.

Many will have been moved by the decision of the Portsmouth diocese in 1985 not to have any synods, committee or PCC meetings during Lent *in order to listen to God*. The results must have been dynamic. Indeed a layman in the diocese witnessed at one of my seminars to the deepening of faith among God's people, while the Provost of the Cathedral told me of the grateful reaction from people outside the churches that at last we were doing our real job! *Si sic omnes!*

The transfiguration of the universe into the Kingdom of God, that is, the place where God's will is done and his name hallowed; the healing of creation through a pilgrim people fed in the totality of their being by the Lord — in a wholesome relationship of mutual forgiveness with each other under God — and seeking guidance for the Way at every step; this is the canvas Jesus gave us for our prayer and work for him, the map for the journey of the People of God on the Way. There is actually some justification for calling it the Prayer of the Kingdom, the prayer purposely designed as the spiritual designation for the People of the Way, 'as John also taught his disciples'. In any case it provides the motivation not only for the journey but for our life-giving relationship with the God-on-ahead. It encapsulates the important matters concerning which we need to have dialogue with God. Above all it is the *Lord's* prayer, a priceless legacy from him, and every time we use it we are at one with him and in him. It is therefore a valuable source of unity and cohesion for his People on the way, seeking to follow him who is the Way.

Emphasis has often been laid on a sense of duty with regard to prayer. As Christians we 'owe' it to God. It would be preferable to think of it in terms of love, the flow of love from God to us and through us back to him. This seemed to be the case when Jesus spent long hours, often before daylight, in communion with his Father. It underlines the need for a desire of the heart as a basic requirement for the two-way process of converse with God which is prayer. And this continual converse with God is the thirst-quenching water for the journey which must flow continually if the journey is to be pursued to the end.

Water is always an important element on a journey. As regards the sheer necessity to have drinking water it is vital (of life). We have seen that the need of the Israelites for drinking water at Marah led to the revelation of their God as Healer. It is therefore necessary to come across streams, springs and rivers on the journey of life, for they have life-giving properties. All these play important parts on the biblical journeys. Of course, water can also be a barrier, as the Israelites found at the Red Sea; and a point of danger, as Peter discovered when he looked down when walking on the water towards Jesus, and as Paul also discovered on his journey to Rome. But for the most part water is seen as an element expressive of salvation and healing, to which the prophets have pointed as the final outcome of the journey.

The prophetic line ends in John the Baptist, who confronts those who come to him with stern teaching about where they are on their journey, preaching a baptism of *metanoia* (repentance). This word has little to do with sackcloth and ashes, but rather means a total change of heart and mind, or, in accord with the metaphor we have been using, a complete U-turn on the journey of life. The experience outside the gates of Damascus which transformed Saul the Zealot into Paul the Apostle was in the first place a *metanoia*. It also points to the second part of the word's meaning — a coming home to God. It is therefore an important element on the journey to wholeness, which is of course ultimately a journey into God. John the Baptist's ministry was a baptism of repentance, confronting people with the need for *metanoia* and then immersing them in the healing waters to enable them to continue on the journey to wholeness clothed with their salvific properties.

Water in the New Testament takes on its greatest dignity when used in Christian baptism. The water of life which Jesus promised to the woman at the well is given by being born again in him, sharing his death and resurrection, in the waters of baptism. Indeed, the feetwashing which the writer of the fourth gospel records on the night before Jesus died, is often seen as an institution of Christian baptism, just as the other Gospel writers record the institution of the Eucharist, the other Gospel sacrament, at that place. These events seem to be sealed in Jesus' death on the cross, when at the piercing of his side, 'blood and water' are seen to flow out, symbolic of the two sacraments, the eucharist and baptism, which are both part of the pilgrim's necessary food and equipment for the journey.

Let us pause and ponder for a moment how health-giving are the two Gospel sacraments, and therefore how *vital* for our journey to wholeness. Baptism has been called the primary healing sacrament, primary because at once it sets in motion the healing of our birth trauma and heals us into the Community of the People of the Way. The whole act centres on the dying and rising again with Christ, symbolized by the going down into the waters (the extinction of life) and the rising up out of them (resurrection). This gives the recipient an experience of the power of the risen Lord and so of his healing. Again, baptism is a new birth, an experience of being born again in body and soul. In it we receive a new wholeness. The potential in our humanity towards illness, brokenness and disintegration, is transformed towards wholeness and integration. It should also be noted that in baptism an exorcism is used, prayers for the deliverance of the child from evil which is an ever more pressing remedy of preventive medicine in today's world; also the laying on of hands, in the healing touch given to the child or candidate. It is also a washing away of sins, a therapy of which all of us are in need; and in the Eastern rite there is an anointing with oil (chrism) 'unto the healing of body and soul'.

This healing property is continued in the Eucharist. As in baptism, there is a forgiveness (absolution) of the past, an opportunity for recalling not only our sins of omission and commission, but also our hurts, resentments and fears, and of surrendering them to Christ present in his 'timeless potency', Bishop Michael Ramsey's phrase. If these latter are left in us to fester, they are liable to rear their ugly heads again in organic disease. The time when the Church recalls the salvific and healing act of Christ in his cross/resurrection is the God-given opportunity for recalling our hurts so that we may receive inner healing of anything we have smothered and repressed into our subconscious mind.

Another dimension of the Eucharist, the food for pilgrims, is that as well as being a sacrament of redemption it is also a sacrament of creation. This is reflected in the ancient offertory prayers we are rightly using again:

Blessed are you, Lord God of all creation. Through your goodness we have this bread to offer, which earth has given and human hands have made. It will become for us the bread of life.

And again:

Blessed are you, Lord God of all creation. Through your goodness we have this wine to offer, fruit of the vine and work of human hands. It will become our spiritual drink.

It is essential for our health that we maintain a close relationship with the soil, and this desire we can consecrate in this 'anticipatory sacrament of a healed creation'.

A few years ago we were talking on these lines in a seminar in Kendal when a lady very humbly declared herself to be a horticultural therapist. She worked on the staff of a mental hospital, where she helped and guided each patient to cultivate their own allotment. She had a resulting personal and therapeutic relationship with them all as she taught them to have a relationship with the soil. There was a gradual improvement in the awareness and mental health of many of them. I was happy to learn that her spiritual base was Carlisle Cathedral where she was, and still is, supported in prayer.

The other dimension of the Eucharist which is therapy for us all is the relationship enjoyed with the whole redeemed community in Christ, 'with angels and archangels and the whole company of heaven'. Here is the right time and place for Christians to have healthy relationships with their dead and with the saints, when all are present in Christ and

Christ is present to all. This is necessary therapeutic teaching which we have been slow to offer.

Here then is the 'blood and water' for ever flowing from his pierced side. By his wounds we are healed indeed. It is the Lamb who leads us on our journey to springs of living water (Rev. 7.17) which flow out from the throne of God and of the Lamb (Rev. 21 and 22). Here in the last chapters of our Bible we find this final vision of John, an exile on the isle of Patmos. He is led to see the Holy City, coming down from God, who also comes finally to live with man so that all death, pain and sickness are finally banished. 'I am making everything new,' proclaims the Alpha and Omega, the Beginning and the End (of our journey), from the throne. Thirst, an inevitable element on the journey, will finally be assuaged 'without cost from the spring of the water of life'.

John is then shown this river of the water of life 'flowing from the throne of God and of the Lamb down the middle of the great street of the city'. He then learns the purpose of this great flow of water: it is for healing. 'On each side of the river stood the tree of life, bearing twelve crops of fruit, yielding its fruit every month. And the leaves of the tree are for the healing of the nations.' The blessed ones are those 'who wash their robes, that they may have the right to the tree of life and may go through the gates into the city'. Always moving on. The journey must be completed. The gates must be entered in order to experience the healing properties of the tree of life. It *is*, after all, a journey to wholeness, and journey's end *is* lovers' meeting.

This water of healing, this vital communication with God, this spring of living water, is beginning again to flow down the middle alley of our churches and Christian communities. We must praise God for the 'new springtime in the Church'. The tap that will keep this flood of healing water flowing in our communities and in ourselves as we journey on together is a flood of prayer. Prayer is the propelling force on the journey. It is also the healing stream that will preserve our bodies and souls so that the journey can be continued. The God-on-ahead is the God who heals.

I first began to realize this when years ago Anne and I happened to change our prayer pattern. We had always said the offices together whenever possible. Now we began to share together our times of contemplative silence. The consequent process of slowing down the whole bodily activity, which can now be measured clinically, led to a slowing down of some of life's rush and tumble and, I suppose, a diminution of stress. The headaches at times of overwork became far less frequent and now seldom occur. This does not mean that we fail to take precautions. We try not to put God to the test! But it is worth recording that this happens to be our experience and I do not for one moment suspect it is unique. In fact, written evidence of prayer as therapy is increasingly forthcoming.

One example is *The Relaxation Response* by Herbert Benson to which I have already referred (Chapter 2). I first met Dr Benson at a conference on new trends in health care at the Royal College of Physicians in London. He was obviously a deeply spiritual person as I found in conversation the evening before his lecture. In his lecture he told how the worst kind of stress was time stress, working against the clock, and especially driving against the clock. The latter is liable to bring stress to countless others also! This he felt was one of the prime causes of bringing people, or more often of people being brought, into his clinic. I can recall the astonished gasp of the audience — mostly physicians from all over the world — when he calmly said that he now more frequently prescribed prayer than drugs. When questioned on this remark at the end of his lecture, he showed how he had studied the prayer forms and spirituality of all the major religions and would try to prescribe the prayer form relevant to a person's belief. For a Christian patient he would most frequently prescribe the Jesus prayer, because he found that the slow repetition of 'Lord Jesus Christ — Son of God — have mercy on me — a sinner' resonated with the heart rhythms and body chemistry most beneficially. I do not think he would advocate prayer solely as a means of avoidance of cardiovascular disease, but his clinical experience is that consistent prayer of a contemplative kind is manifestly therapeutic.

This leads to interesting speculation concerning the hermits and monks of olden times. When one sees the magnificent ruins of some monasteries, invariably built by or over water making them even more cold, one is led to wonder how they survived, especially from being totally frozen in the vigils of the night. Perhaps the altered states of consciousness induced by the regular round of prayer and contemplation had something to do, not only with the survival but also with the flourishing, of the monasteries for so many centuries. Their discipline of prayer and work certainly produced a hardy breed.

Yet another factor in the 'health' of the monasteries was the fact that they were living systems. The secret of their communal life was that it was an interconnected and integrated whole at every point. The central link in the whole system was the Church and all it stood for, which gave purpose and motivation to all that went on in the total life of the community. It was the corporate round of prayer, shared by all, day and night, with the differing moods of the various seasons and festivals, that directed the life of the system Godward, and so aligned the whole into his will.

The monastic life today may have been decimated numerically, but the general impression given to those of us outside it is of a renewed spiritual strength and relevance to the world situation. Indeed the number of those in secular life who have some connection with conventual life, by a shared rule or through making retreats and being under the spiritual guidance of a religious, may well be increasing. Is this a yearning of the Church, at this point in its journey, to become increasingly the community of Christ, the fellowship of the Holy Spirit, centred in the life of the blessed Trinity? Is this a realization of the right time (*ho kairos*) truly to become the healing community, not only in response to the obvious need of the world but also as an act of obedience to God's call? It seems that the call of the God-on-ahead to the Patriarchs to become a holy nation, the call by Christ — the Alpha and Omega, and similarly therefore calling us from 'beyond' our journey — to be his own to whom he has given his new lifestyle of love and for whom he has died and risen again, and the inner compulsion of the Holy Spirit who sheds this love abroad in our hearts, is being heard and deeply felt in our time. All appearances would seem to be to the contrary when we look at the world scene solely through the eyes of the media and the statisticians. But the gut conviction remains that God is doing an ever-deepening, often cathartic, sometimes miraculous, always sign-giving, work in our time, recalling his own to be what he called them out on the journey to become, 'a chosen people, a royal priesthood, a holy nation, a people belonging to God' (1 Peter 2.9).

At this stage on its journey we seem to be witnessing the de-privatization of the Church in more senses than one. The

Church had allowed itself to be pushed on to the confines of society, getting on with its religion while the state and other organizations took over the welfare of the people and directed their journey. Most people had accepted this, many within the Church, and liked to have it so. The secular (so-called) world had grown up, and having come of age had removed itself from the sacred (so-called) hearth. Once again, however, we are hearing prophetic voices — and possibly even more powerfully experiencing a new life within the Christian community — that are together calling the people of God to move on and out into the next stage of their journey, to be with the Christ-on-ahead in the centre of the world he came to redeem. Christianity is not for the Church but for the world. If we allow it to become the preserve of the Church alone we privatize it and opt out of the journey on which we are called to travel. This all seems so obvious, but privatization has happened in our time. Now we are seeing the signs of a moving on as the journey again gets under way.

There is an implication here for each of us individually, for personal religion had also become privatized. The God-on-ahead calls to his whole people and is now calling all his people into a new wholeness. His call comes to his community to be his holy people. There is invariably a corporateness about his call to traverse the journey. We owe it to him that we do not permit this call to become privatized, individualized, again. The call comes to us *within community*. And even if we are conscious of that call individually, we shall soon discover that God has been saying the same things to others within the community at the same time. We shall find that what we deemed to be an individual call has a dynamic corporateness about it.

In a time of sharing with seventy Baptist ministers I was interested to hear how they were expressing their consciousness and that of their congregations in terms of the healing community. I have since then frequently heard the expression of such a consciousness right across the Christian spectrum and beyond, for I have heard such ideas expressed in hospitals and schools. This need not be such a strange idea as it first might seem. What is a community of people called to live and work and serve together but a community of healing, both as regards the members of the community themselves and also all who enter or pass through that community? How can any community, be it a nuclear family, hospital, board room or church, stay together unless there is not only a unity of purpose but also a growing feeling of solidarity and mutual support which upholds the whole enterprise on the journey forward together? How can the Christian family answer the call to engage in that journey without the love of God being shed abroad in every heart by the Holy Spirit? How can it otherwise join in the whole enterprise of God, which is to establish his reign and so bring about a healed creation? Must it not so lose its life in this world that the whole life of the world is gathered up into the fullness and wholeness of God? Is not the kingdom of this world to become the kingdom of our God and of his Christ? Journey's end is to be lovers' meeting, when the whole creation's travail is fulfilled in the bringing to birth of a new creation, whose only ethic is love.

Could therefore the concept of the Church as the healing community be the figure and sign for our time, for our particular *krisis* on the journey to wholeness? If this could be so, what is the essence of such a community? The word used by Paul and by Luke in Acts is *koinonia* which means communion, fellowship, participation. In classical Greek it meant the unbroken fellowship between the gods and men, but was also applied to the brotherly union between men.

In a Greek version of the Old Testament the word was not used to refer to the relationship between God and man, which was rather referred to in terms of distance (servanthood or covenant), reflecting the Jewish consciousness of the primeval rupture of fellowship with God, who nevertheless constantly attempted to restore this state of fellowship.

In the New Testament there is a distinct change of emphasis. Jesus has come to restore that fellowship with God. The Johannine writer reflects this shift of emphasis in figures like the vine and the flock. Paul and Luke in Acts use the word *koinonia*, as the Greeks did, to denote fellowship with God, which in the Christian dispensation is through or with Jesus Christ in the unity of the Holy Spirit. The primary fellowship is on the vertical plane therefore: 'God, who has called you into fellowship with his Son Jesus Christ our Lord . . .' (1 Cor. 1.9); but it is also reflected on the horizontal plane: 'They devoted themselves to the apostles' teaching and to the fellowship, to the breaking of bread and to prayer' (Acts 2.42). Even in this latter case it has a possible liturgical significance (cf. 1 Cor. 10.16), and so refers to the fellowship we enjoy with Christ in the Eucharist and so through him with our fellow Christians. But there is one significant difference from the Greek usage; whereas the Greeks looked back to a golden age of sharing, Christians look forward to the time of sharing with their Lord and each other in the eschatological banquet in the Kingdom of God. Christians are therefore people who are on the Way, their whole attention fixed on him who is the Way, watching, waiting, alert for his coming. The fellowship they enjoy with Christ means for them a birth into a new existence, a process of transfiguration through incorporation into the dying and rising again of Christ, a journey from death to life, a participation in the eschatological community of God.

The healing community is that which is in process of being healed because the God who heals has his hand upon it, while according to his promise, Jesus is in the midst. That is why it is the fellowship of the Holy Spirit. Privilege, however, brings obligations and the obligations we are under are *to watch* (wait and listen), *to 'do this'*, (the Eucharist), and *to love*. This is the essential travel equipment of the healing community, for they are the direct commands of Jesus to his disciples.

1. *Watch.* I remember being told in my early days, 'If you only have five minutes to pray, spend four of them in silent waiting upon God.' It is not a bad ratio, not only for the spiritual life but for the whole life of the healing community. Our deep sin is that we rush around in phrenetic activity doing good and working for the Church (*sic*) in a totally undirected and unguided, too often misguided, way. When do we place every deed and word under the scrutiny and direction of God? How much honest listening to God is on our personal or ecclesial agenda? I know from my own experience, even having seen the desperate need to perceive and wait upon the Lord's will in every situation, that it is negligible. We will go bashing along the road without waiting for his green light.

There has undoubtedly been a turning again to prayer by all sections of the churches in recent times. I do not mean to say that the Church has ever given up on prayer, but there has been of late, possibly mainly thanks to the renewal movement, a noticeable increase in groups of Christians praying together. This has been the largest single factor in the renewal of the vitality of the Christian Church in many places. But these very groups

103

of Christians have tended, often because of their new found faith, to become noisier and, quite rightly, louder in singing God's praises, but without the essential balance of long silence in order to listen to the Lord who is longing to speak to them, if they have ears to hear. How vital for any fellowship that would be part of God's healing community is the silence of waiting. It is the essential preparation for setting out on the Way. It is the essential run-in to any synod, for does not that word mean those who go together on the Way? A synod should be composed of those who so travel together that they are waiting for instructions concerning their every step from the God-on-ahead who summons them to venture forward together on *his* way, his journey to wholeness.

How right was Bishop Festo Kivengere of Uganda when he said: 'Prayer is not just a flood of words. Prayer is when a person goes out of himself or herself and steps into the presence of God. This is never easy.' Yes, it is never easy to set out on the journey. It is hard to leave the flood of words behind. It is so much easier to cover up the silence with noise. But the stepping forward on the journey in prayerful faith in order to enter the presence of God is the object of the journey. And that journey can only be complete in his presence.

2. *Do this.* It is essential therefore that we have food for the way, as the Israelites had manna in the wilderness. God has supplied this in the 'bread of the world in mercy broken', the pilgrim food in the Eucharist, the corporate meal of the healing community on the Way. Alexander Schmemann described it in terms of the journey: 'The Eucharist is the journey of the Church into the dimension of the Kingdom . . . the holding of the past

and future in the now of faith.' It is an entering into the sphere of God's presence and reign so that the community is enfolded in his will. There is a focus of timelessness in the 'now of faith'.

St Irenaeus, at the beginning of the Christian era, also perceived its healing properties: 'The power of the Eucharist gives life to the body as well as the soul.' A similar thought was expressed in the Liturgy of St Basil 'for the welfare and sanctification and healing of our souls and bodies', as well as in the Book of Common Prayer, both in the prayer of humble access and in the first words of administration, ' . . . preserve thy body and soul unto everlasting life'. It is the healing balm for the healing community on its journey to wholeness.

3. *Love.* The third piece of equipment is love, greater even than faith and hope, because it is of God, and 'God is love' (1 John 4.8). And so 'If I speak in the tongues of men and of angels, but have not love, I am only a resounding gong or a clanging cymbal' (1 Cor. 13.1). Love is the first fruit of the Spirit (Gal. 5.22). It is the area in which to seek primary growth in the healing community, for it speaks wholly of God. The absence of blossom or fruit in this area is an indication of a lack of healing and a lack of community.

Love is no soft option. It is a journey of the will, in tune with the God of love, towards the total good of the other. It was the new commandment that Jesus laid on his disciples the night before he set out on his salvific journey of death and resurrection. It is therefore his last will and testament to all who would follow him.

Too often the healing community's journey, and its effectiveness, is atrophied by lack of love, by harmful relationships which speak to the outsider, or to one who comes newly in, of unhealing. All of us have known this, most of us at first hand because we have been part of that unhealed situation. There is nothing that so quickly destroys God's work as a condition of unhealing or disease in the Body of Christ, just as any malfunction or disease will destroy the wholesome working of the human body. We have to allow the healing streams of God's love to irrigate all relationships within the healing community. We also have to co-operate with his healing love by allowing it to activate our will in order to be positive in our love for each individual in the community and for the total good of the whole community. This will involve a constant setting out from where we are now: an ever new willingness to say our 'Amen' to the Lord's invitation to journey towards him; for the closer our relationship to him, the more loving will be our relationship with each other. But it does mean movement, because to be nearer to him and to each other it is we who have to do the travelling and move on, in order to become his healing community.

It was the Holy Spirit of Movement who drove Jesus into the wilderness to preface his own journey with that period of waiting upon the Father's will. The Spirit is the driving force, visualized by the apostles under the forms of two powerful elements, wind and fire, the power that motivates the healing community on its journey to wholeness. There is no preconceived map for that journey. It will be uncharted and different territory for each one of us. The constant need is to set out, and even when, or perhaps especially when, the Temple is in good order, to take the sacrificial option of the Tent and say our 'Amen' to the Lord's invitation to go for him, as his community on the road. As we listen to him and keep sensitive to his bidding

106

as he unfolds to us our eternal destiny, we shall experience his food of love. It is the timelessness of that destiny and of the journey towards its discovery that forms the seedbed for this fruit of love. And love is the motive power behind all our travelling, for it is redolent with the fire of the Spirit.

This means that the travelling must be together, in God and in each other, for journey's end is lovers' meeting. The seer of Patmos' vision of this was the Holy City, the divine community whose centre is the throne of God and of the Lamb, whence flow the healing waters. The refreshment of journey's end will be to be washed in these waters which irrigate the trees whose leaves are for the healing of the nations. Our self-centredness, individual and corporate, will be absorbed into the mercy and love of God as all are healed into the divine community. As St Augustine put it, we shall rest and we shall see, we shall see and we shall love, we shall love and we shall praise — in the knowledge that we were called on a journey to the wholeness that is in God alone, into 'the silence of eternity, interpreted by love'. Or, as T. S. Eliot so movingly wrote of man's quest,

> With the drawing of this Love and the voice of this
>   Calling.
> We shall not cease from exploration,
> And the end of all our exploring
> Will be to arrive where we started
> And to know the place for the first time.[1]

APPENDIX

The Acorn Christian Healing Trust

Together with four Trustees, Anne and I founded the Trust in April 1983 to support our work and develop the initiatives we were taking on my appointment as Adviser to the Archbishops of Canterbury and York. Throughout its history the Trust has relied on the generosity of trusts, parishes and individuals as well as the hard work of the Trustees.

Our objectives have been:

1. *To encourage the working together of the churches centrally and locally in health and healing activities.* To this end we have encouraged all the Church of England bishops, many Roman Catholic bishops and the Free Church leaders to appoint advisers and we have provided their training. Archdeacon Trevor Nash is the staff member responsible for this side of the work.
2. *To develop co-operation between the Church and Medicine at all levels, especially in the local situation.* On our travels we have recruited pairs of Christians, one of whom has been medically trained, to act as a sign of the healing Christ in their hospital, surgery, parish, etc., and to take initiatives for the Kingdom. We have named them the *Acorn Apostolate*. Anne and I lead this part of the work. Bonded together by regular weekend courses and an annual conference, they have set up many initiatives including Christian Cancer Help Centres, homes of healing and peace, places of teaching and training, of care for the mentally sick and of listening.
3. *To promote the healing ministry through training in listening,*

in which Church and Medicine may also co-operate. We recruited our first member of staff, the Reverend Anne Long, in January 1985 to develop this side of the work. She has pioneered the teaching and training of *Christian Listeners,* assisted by several staff members including the Reverend Russ Parker, our deputy. It has become such a large part of the work that it is undergoing a major overhaul of its administration. Christian Listeners are active in schools, prisons, hospitals, surgeries as well as in all the main churches. They are now being used in Cathedrals.

4. *To provide a resource of teaching and training in the Christian healing ministry.* The Acorn Trust has found a generous friend in the Whitehill Chase Foundation Trust, which has provided us with a headquarters and resource centre (Whitehill Chase, Bordon, GU35 0AP) in Hampshire together with a fine chapel and conference room. Teaching, training and healing retreat conferences are held here. Canon Stephen Sidebotham and his wife Peggy head an efficient and willing staff which include the Administrator Jamie Jamieson and his wife Gwen. There is also a large voluntary team.

The Trustees are headed by Charles Longbottom and include two doctors, a Cathedral Provost and a Canon of another Cathedral, a Roman Catholic peer, a banker and businessmen. The Trust won the Templeton (UK) award for 1994. The Archbishop of Canterbury has asked the Trust to work closely with his own Springboard initiative for the decade of evangelism. Tasks and targets are set by the staff and undertaken for the glory of God and his Kingdom with an emphasis on good communication between all engaged in the Lord's work of Christian Healing.

Notes

Chapter 1   **Preparing for the Journey**

1. The late Dr Evans, who was Dean of Salisbury, offered this definition in his inaugural lecture to the 'Health for the Eighties' Conference at Swanwick in 1981, organized by the Churches' Council for Health and Healing.
2. This is one reason why the high rise flats have been a disaster.
3. In this book I have used both alternative spellings, 'wholistic' and 'holistic'. I prefer the former, as better expressing the concept of wholeness, but have sometimes retained the latter as it is commonly used with reference to the holistic movement in medicine.
4. For instance, normally human beings have a cerebral cortex measuring 4.5 centimetres in thickness, containing 15 to 20 billion neurons, some of which are capable of firing twenty times per second. The synaptic cleft (the junction between neurons), in which quantum phenomena are known to operate, is never quiet. Some scientists think this wave activity enables the brain to encode information holographically. See Larry Dossey, M.D., *Space, Time and Medicine* (Shambhala, Boulder and London, 1982) pp. 106–10.

Chapter 2   **A Biblical Pilgrimage**

1. It is of interest that one of the archetypes which C. G. Jung sees as significant in what he calls the process of individuation, a process which has many points in common with our journey to wholeness, is that of the child as the symbol of hidden potential, of hope through marvellous growth. A myth about the birth of a wonderful child is to be found in many cultures. In these stories

the child is exposed to great hazards surrounding its birth but, strangely protected and delivered from extreme dangers, is enabled to grow to its full potential and complete its 'journey'. The story of Hercules in mythology is an obvious example, but the prime examples in the Bible are Moses and Jesus himself. Both were born in places of great hardship, both lives were sought by murderous monarchs, both had to survive if the journey of God's people was to continue. (We should also notice in passing the part women played in God's plan of salvation, like Mary the mother of Jesus; even the king's daughter played a part in the saving of Moses.) By this process of individuation, Jung meant a movement of maturing growth and human development which proceeds side by side with biological growth until the individual is mature enough to participate in the process in order to complete it. By the archetype, an inherited tendency closely allied to instinct, Jung meant the choosing principle in each of us by which we respond to certain stimuli and not to others. Jung has much to contribute to our quest for spiritual maturity and to our equipment for the journey.

2. See Kosuke Koyama, *Three Mile an Hour God* (SCM Press 1979) chapter 1.
3. Hans Kung, *On Being a Christian* (Collins 1977) p. 231.

Chapter 3 **A Medical Pilgrimage**

1. Fritjof Capra, *The Turning Point* (Fontana 1983) p. 337f.
2. op. cit., p. 343.
3. Herbert Benson, *The Relaxation Response* (Fount 1984).

Chapter 4 **In Search of a Vision**

1. R. A. Butler in *The Art of Memory* recalls a Churchillian tour of

English history as the great man gazed across the Weald of Kent from this seat of meditation.

2. See Norman Perrin, *The Kingdom of God in the Teaching of Jesus* (SCM Press 1963) chapter 10. I am indebted to his thinking about the Kingdom.
3. Kenneth Kirk, *The Vision of God* (James Clarke 1977).
4. e.g. Gerhard von Rad, quoted and supported by Norman Perrin.
5. A thought from Rowan Williams, *The Wound of Knowledge* (Darton, Longman and Todd 1979).
6. Austin Farrer, *The Revelation of St John the Divine* (Oxford University Press 1964) p. 28.
7. Frank Wright, *The Pastoral Nature of the Ministry* (SCM Press 1980). See especially chapters 2–4.
8. I am grateful to my colleague the Rev. Dr Roy Walford for pointing out the common derivation of the words religion and ligaments. The latter are the flexible tissue that services the joints and holds them in place!

Chapter 6 **The People of the Way Move On**

1. In *The Christian Healing Ministry* (SPCK 1981) chapter 6.
2. See Resolution 8 of Lambeth XI (1978) and the report of Lambeth XII (1988) entitled 'The Truth Shall Make You Free', pp. 47–9.
3. He died in October 1944 and though the free world was engaged in fighting for its life in Europe and the Far East, the shock was felt throughout the English-speaking world.
4. For other initiatives see Appendix.
5. David Enoch, *Healing the Hurt Mind* (Hodder 1983).
6. Kenneth Leech, *True God* (Sheldon Press 1985) p. 96.
7. Ibid. p. 97.

Chapter 7 **Journey's End is Lovers' Meeting**

1. T. S. Eliot, *Little Gidding* (Collected Poems 1909–1962).